Plant-derived Hepatoprotective Drugs

Edited by

Sachin Kumar Jain
Oriental College of Pharmacy & Research, Oriental University
Opp. Rewati Range Sanwer Road Indore
MP 453555, India

Ram Kumar Sahu
Department of Pharmaceutical Sciences,
Hemvati Nandan Bahuguna Garhwal University (A Central University), Chauras Campus
Tehri Garhwal-249161,
Uttarakhand, India

Priyanka Soni
B R Nahata College of Pharmacy
Mandsaur University
Mandsaur,
India

Vishal Soni
B R Nahata College of Pharmacy
Mandsaur University
Mandsaur,
India

&

Shiv Shankar Shukla
Columbia Institute of Pharmacy
Tekri Raipur,
India

Plant-derived Hepatoprotective Drugs

Editors: Sachin Kumar Jain, Ram Kumar Sahu, Priyanka Soni, Vishal Soni and Shiv Shankar Shukla

ISBN (Online): 978-981-5079-84-5

ISBN (Print): 978-981-5079-85-2

ISBN (Paperback): 978-981-5079-86-9

need for a court order if at any point you breach any terms of this License Agreement. In no event will any delay or failure by Bentham Science Publishers in enforcing your compliance with this License Agreement constitute a waiver of any of its rights.

3. You acknowledge that you have read this License Agreement, and agree to be bound by its terms and conditions. To the extent that any other terms and conditions presented on any website of Bentham Science Publishers conflict with, or are inconsistent with, the terms and conditions set out in this License Agreement, you acknowledge that the terms and conditions set out in this License Agreement shall prevail.

Bentham Science Publishers Pte. Ltd.
80 Robinson Road #02-00
Singapore 068898
Singapore
Email: subscriptions@benthamscience.net

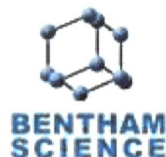

**BENTHAM
SCIENCE**

CONTENTS

PREFACE

Since the ancient period, plants have shown a pivotal role in leading a healthy life. In developing countries, plant based medicines have great importance to the people. Herbal medicines are used for the treatment of liver diseases for an extended time. The Liver, is the foremost organ for maintaining the human body's internal surroundings. Its major influence is on the flow of nutrients and controls the metabolism of carbohydrates, macromolecule and fats.

The book is an exclusive version of instructive matter in the aspect of Plant Derived Hepatoprotectives, a compilation of ten excellent review articles presenting the latest development in this field of natural product services. They cover a wide range of topics, all relevant to the evidence based therapeutic, protective and olfactory uses of common herbs.

The review by Ikbal *et al.* is focused on the anatomy, functions of the liver, types of liver injury, risk factors and various treatment strategies for liver diseases. Toxicology of the liver is a complex concept that entails either concurrent as well as sequential events. Drug-induced liver injury to the liver can match any form of acute or chronic liver injury. In the next review, the authors have highlighted the various hepatoprotective roles of medicinal plants. Details of Bioactive components and mode of action of hepatoprotective activity of the medicinal plant. With fewer side effects, herbal drugs have gained much attention in the mitigation of various liver disorders and in maintaining a healthy life. The author has provided a comprehensive chapter covering the scientific hepatoprotective agents that are often the treatment of choice to improve liver function and protect the liver from exposure to harmful compounds. Impressive studies have exposed that the health-promoting outcomes of bioactive constituents derivated from plants have often been applied to their antioxidant characteristics and raise cellular antioxidant protection system, scavenge free radicals, suppress lipid peroxidation, stimulate anti-inflammatory capacity, and assure the liver from destruction. These compounds are chlorogenic acid, curcumin, quercetin, hesperidin, rutin, betalains, apigenin, sylimarin, phyllanthin, mangiferin, α-mangostin, bellidifolin, ginsenosides, glycyrrhizin, lycopene, and andrographolide. Anishma*et al* has contributed a chapter on hepatoprotective effect of flavonoids. Many of the flavonoids have hepatoprotective activity and they are been used in traditional medicine to treat any kind of diseases like liver dysfunction and other damages caused by hepatoprotective. The next review by Jain NK and Singh N is also focused on various hepatoprotective plants and herbal formulations. Authors compile information on promising phytochemicals from medicinal plants that have been tested in hepatotoxicity models using cutting-edge scientific methods.

The next review by Jha *et al.* is also focused on the Regulatory affairs in herbal products. The review focused on various parameters/guidelines regulating the safety and efficacy of herbal pharmaceuticals, as well as their manufacturing and distribution, which have been strongly implemented by regulatory bodies. This chapter covers the importance of regulatory affairs to be used in the processing of herbs and herbal products and a comparative study of regulatory situations in different countries. Chakraborty R and Sen S have written a chapter on Hepatoprotective effects of edible plants and spices. The author focused on as part of the diet, edible plants could play an important role in protecting the liver from injury caused by oxidative stress, microorganism, or other exogenous substances This chapter highlighted edible plants with hepatoprotective activity. Koka SS *et al.* discuss the the role of terpenoids as hepatoprotective. Plants with a high level of terpenoids appear to have good hepatoprotective properties. Sweta S Koka *et al.* focused on the hepatoprotective effect of the tannin-rich compound. The tannin-containing drugs suppress or inhibit the formation of free radicals generated due to the metabolism of hepato-toxins. Tannins are widely used in marketed formulations that are used in the treatment of hepato-toxicity. The next review by Sarkar BK presented a chapter on hepatoprotective phytochemicals: isolation and characterization from plant extracts. The author has presented the advances in phytochemistry. The authors have presented the advance in phytochemistry and the number of herbal and herbomineral preparations available in the Ayurveda, the traditional Indian Medicine which, have been investigated for its hepatoprotective potential to treat different types of liver disorders. The present review is focused on different herbal plants that have the potential to cure hepatotoxicity.

Sachin Kumar Jain
Oriental College of Pharmacy & Research, Oriental University
Opp. Rewati Range Sanwer Road Indore
MP 453555, India

Ram Kumar Sahu
Department of Pharmaceutical Sciences
Hemvati Nandan Bahuguna Garhwal University (A Central University), Chauras
Campus
Tehri Garhwal-249161,
Uttarakhand, India

Priyanka Soni
B R Nahata College of Pharmacy
Mandsaur University
Mandsaur,
India

Vishal Soni
B R Nahata College of Pharmacy
Mandsaur University
Mandsaur,
India

&

Shiv Shankar Shukla
Columbia Institute of Pharmacy
Tekri Raipur,
India

List of Contributors

Abu Md Ashif Ikbal   Department of Pharmaceutical Sciences, Assam University (A Central University), Silchar -788011, Assam, India

Bedanta Bhattacharjee   Department of Pharmaceutical Sciences, Faculty of Science and Engineering, Dibrugarh University, Dibrugarh-786004, Assam, India

Biresh Kumar Sarkar   Central Ayurveda Research Institute, CCRAS, Ministry of AYUSH, 4-CN Block, Sector- V, Bidhannagar, Kolkata- 700091, India

Deepshikha Verma   Institute of Pharmaceutical Sciences, Guru Ghasidas Vishwavidyalaya (A Central University), Koni, Bilaspur-495009, Chhattisgarh, India

Dhrubajyoti Sarkar   Faculty of Pharmaceutical Science, Assam Down town University Sankar Medhab Path Panikhaiti Guwahati 781026, India

Dolly Rani   Amity Institutes of Pharmacy, Amity University, Noida-201303, India

Durgaprasad Kemisetti   Faculty of Pharmaceutical Science, Assam Down Town University, Panikhaiti, Guwahati, Assam- 781026, India

Faruk Alam   Faculty of Pharmaceutical Science, Assam Down Town University, Panikhaiti, Guwahati, Assam- 781026, India

Kavita Chahal   Department of Botany, Government College, Chhindwara, M.P. 480111, India

Megha Jha   Department of Research, Pinnacle Biomedical Research Institute, Bhopal, M.P. 462003, India

Monika Kaurav   KIET School of Pharmacy, KIET Groups of Institutions, Delhi-NCR, Meerut Road (NH-58) Ghaziabad – 201206, India

Neetesh Kumar Jain   Department of Pharmacology, Modern Institute of Pharmaceutical Sciences, Indore, MP, India

Nitu Singh   RGS College of Pharmacy, Itaunja, Lucknow, UP, India

Parikshit Das   Department of Pharmaceutical Sciences, Assam University (A Central University), Silchar-788011, Assam, India

Paromita Dutta Choudhury   Department of Pharmaceutical Sciences, Assam University (A Central University), Silchar-788011, Assam, India

Raja Chakraborty   Institute of Pharmacy, Assam Don Bosco University, Tapesia Gardens, Sonapur – 782 402, Assam, India

Ram Kumar Sahu   Department of Pharmaceutical Sciences, Hemvati Nandan Bahuguna Garhwal University (A Central University), Chauras Campus, Tehri Garhwal-249161, Uttarakhand, India

Retno Widyowati   Department of Pharmaceutical Science, Faculty of Pharmacy, Universitas Airlangga, Surabaya, 60115, Indonesia

Rosita Handayani   Natural Product Drug Discovery and Development Research Group, Faculty of Pharmacy, Universitas Airlangga, Surabaya, 60115, Indonesia

Sachin Kumar Jain   Oriental College of Pharmacy & Research, Oriental University Opp. Rewati Range Sanwer Road, Indore MP 453555, India

Saikat Sen   Faculty of Pharmaceutical Science, Assam down town University, Guwahati, Assam, india

Saket Singh Chandel   Department of Pharmacology, Dr. C. V. Raman Institute of Pharmacy, Dr. C. V. Raman University, Bilaspur-495113, Chhattisgarh, India

Tirna Paul   Department of Pharmaceutical Sciences, Faculty of Science and Engineering, Dibrugarh University, Dibrugarh-786004, Assam, India

CHAPTER 1

Hepatotoxicity

Abu Md Ashif Ikbal[1], Parikshit Das[1], Saket Singh Chandel[2,*], Deepshikha Verma[3] and Paromita Dutta Choudhury[1]

[1] *Department of Pharmaceutical Sciences, Assam University (A Central University), Silchar-788011, Assam, India*

[2] *Department of Pharmacology, Dr. C.V. Raman Institute of Pharmacy, Dr. C. V. Raman University, Bilaspur-495113, Chhattisgarh, India*

[3] *Institute of Pharmaceutical Sciences, Guru Ghasidas Vishwavidyalaya (A Central University), Koni, Bilaspur-495009, Chhattisgarh, India*

Abstract: The largest organ in the human body is the liver which captures 2 to 3% of the human body weight, located on the right side of the anterior quadrant in the abdomen and below the anterior hemidiaphragm ribcage. It performs various important functions such as digestion of food, protein production, fluid production, detoxification of waste, *etc*. Liver injury known as liver trauma can be categorized into four types: hepatocellular, autoimmune, cholestatic and infiltrative. Drug-induced liver injury can match with any form of acute or chronic liver injury. Acute injury to the liver is mainly due to the action of cytochrome P450, which disintegrates drugs into electrophiles or free radicals; these reactive metabolites can covalently act on protein and unsaturated fatty acids for induction of lipid peroxidation which leads to calcium homeostasis or death. Toxicology of the liver is a complex concept that entails either concurrent as well as sequential events. These events determine the pathways, severity and effects of liver injury. Pharmacogenetics has made great progress in current years which indicates the creation of refined algorithms that take drug, host and environmental risk variables into account, allowing for the selection of better medicine based on accurate risk-benefit ratio calculations. In this chapter, we will discuss the anatomy, functions of the liver, types of liver injury, risk factors, and various treatment strategies for the treatment of liver diseases.

Keywords: Cytochrome P450, Hepatocellular, Injury, Liver, Risk factors.

INTRODUCTION

The liver occupies 2 to 3% of the average human body weight thus it is known as the largest organ. The word liver has its meaning rooted in Proto-Germanic "librn", meaning secreting organ of the body (from the source of Old Norse life).

* **Corresponding author Saket Singh Chandel:** Department of Pharmacology, Dr. C.V. Raman Institute of Pharmacy, Dr. C.V. Raman University, Bilaspur-495113, Chhattisgarh, India; Email: singhpharma@gmail.com

Sachin Kumar Jain, Ram Kumar Sahu, Priyanka Soni, Vishal Soni & Shiv Shankar Shukla (Eds.)

It is found in the upper quadrant to the right side of the abdomen under the right hemidiaphragm ribcage that protects it by peritoneal reflection. The place from where it is protected is also known as ligamentous attachments. The ligaments are false and the avascular attachment is in connection with the capsule which is also known as the Glisson capsule [1]. The ligamentous attachment in connection with the umbilical fissure is connected with the falciparum ligament that comes around the umbilicus and extends to the ventral aspect of the liver [2]. There are two lobes present in the liver. The cone-shaped liver also supplies and acquires blood from the sources.

One is the blood that flows from the hepatic artery that is oxygenated and the other is from the hepatic portal vein which is rich in nutrients. At any given point in time, the largest organ can carry blood supply up to one pint (13%) of the total body. The two lobes which are present among the small lobes have eight segments that comprise 1000 lobules. They form a common hepatic duct by linking up the lobules to a small duct that produces a connection to the larger duct.

The only organ that is developed in a vertebrate is the liver [3]. It digests the food we eat and helps in restoring energy and the excretion of toxic substances [4]. Nerves celiac ganglia and vagus nerve are also present in the liver. It is a multitasking organ – the liver is half-moon-shaped, straight and slightly tilted in the cavity of the body. The right portion lies at the initial portion of the small intestine and the left portion is above the stomach. The liver also is the only organ that can regenerate itself as it can replace its parts after 12 partial liver removal surgeries. It is a vascular organ: liver lobule has 3 structures. Each structure can be found in the respective corner of its portal vein, hexagon bile duct and hepatic artery. The blood flow is about 1500ml/min which is approximately about 25% of the cardiac output in which the amount is equivalent to a quarter of the blood that the heart pumps. When the liver tissue was observed under a microscope, it looked somewhat like a honeycomb that was organized beautifully.

FUNCTION

The liver is a vital organ [5]. It has many functions in which some of which are mentioned below:

1. Protein production: One of the important proteins that regulate fluids in the bloodstream and avoid sticking to the nearby tissues.

2. Hormones: It carries hormones throughout the body.

3. Fluid Production: Bile that is produced in the liver and stored in the gallbladder helps in digestion, and in the breakdown of fats into fatty acids, which in turn are taken into the body by the digestive tract.

4. Blood: There are a lot of toxins, by-products and harmful substances in a human body. The liver plays a role in filtering out all the blood that passes through the stomach and intestines.

5. Amino acids: Amino acids are responsible for several cellular metabolisms, the synthesis of nucleotides and lipids as well as detoxification reactions.

6. Blood clotting: Important blood clotting coagulants are created from vitamin K. The liver produces bile that helps in the absorption of vitamin K [6].

7. Vitamins and Minerals: The liver is the starting site for an abundant amount of vitamin A, D, E, K and B12. It also stores nutrients like iron and copper.

8. Glucose: In storing glycogen, the liver plays a major role as it removes the glucose from the bloodstream which is not needed.

9. Detoxification: It is an important role and the liver can excrete endogenous and exogenous waste. It also removes waste products such as bilirubin, ammonia and ketones. Afterwards, it converts them into recycling nutrients which can be excreted through feces or urine.

TYPES OF LIVER INJURY

A liver injury is sometimes referred to as liver trauma that can be defined as one form of damage in the liver that constitutes around 5% of all traumas, thus making it the most commonly found abdominal injury. In general, there are four major classes of liver injury which are cholestatic, hepatocellular, autoimmune and infiltrative. Drug-induced liver injury is relatively less common as compared to other disorders but it remains a challenging clinical trouble concerning both diagnosis and management [7].

A drug-induced liver injury is observed in 3-5% of patients who were referred to the hospitals with jaundice [8]. Therefore, it is regarded as the leading cause of acute liver failure in most Western nations, accounting for more than 50% of occurrences [9]. To date, there are no clear diagnostic standards for drug-induced liver injury while the most common procedures performed to determine the etiology of liver injury include liver biopsy and imaging as well as serologic indicators. Thus, direct or idiosyncratic drug-induced liver damage can be identified.

Substances that are innately damaging or toxic to the liver can cause direct hepatotoxicity in humans. A dose-dependent and predictable damage can be reproduced in animals. There is only a 1-to-5-day latency period post administration of large therapeutic or subtherapeutic doses such as in the case of an accidental or purposeful overdose [10, 11].

Direct Hepatoxicity

A condition in which a patient is not suffering from jaundice but still has an elevated levels of serum enzymes is considered as the most important type of direct drug-induced liver injury. This is when the levels of alanine aminotransferase and alkaline phosphatase are elevated, hyperbilirubinemia is not present and symptoms are minimal or nonexistent. Once the medication is stopped or the advised dose is reduced the increases will reduce as well.

One of the most common forms of clinically apparent direct liver toxicity, acute hepatic necrosis occurs almost always immediately after the medicine is started and more precisely after receiving a single large dose. This kind of ischemic hepatitis is comparable in histology to centrilobular or pan lobular necrosis with minimal inflammation. Untreated acute hepatic necrosis can be fatal; however, the recovery is swift and serum enzyme levels fall as quickly as they rise. This is due to increased dosages of paracetamol, aspirin, nicotinic acid, amiodarone and other anticancer drugs [12, 13]. To begin with, these medications should be administered in low doses.

Idiosyncratic Hepatoxicity

One of the most common signs of idiosyncratic liver injury is acute hepatocellular hepatitis [14, 15]. In histological examinations, eosinophils are prominent thus imply severe viral hepatitis as the significant condition in the variable diagnosis. The fatality rate from icteric hepatocellular injury that is caused by mediators is significant, typically 10% or higher. Due to the fact that this trait had first been observed by the late Hyman J. Zimmerman, it is now commonly known as Hy's Law [16].

As a relatively rare but clinically relevant kind of liver disease, drug-induced liver injury is influenced by how often medications are used and their likelihood of causing injury. Due to how different agents can cause different forms of harm, it poses difficulty to diagnose it.

ANATOMY

Claude Chouinard who was a popular anatomist and physician in 1950, had studied the segmented structure microscopic and macroscopic of the largest gland of the human body *i.e.*, liver. For any hepatic surgeries, the recognitions of the various sections of liver are the utmost requirements. Scientists had examined the internal part of the organ and found that vascular and biliary relationships were based on hepatic functional anatomy [17]. Liver is the largest organ that consists of two lobes which are placed at the right side of the upper quadrant of abdominal cavity [18].

The frontal part of the liver which is connected with an opening named umbilical fissure is continued with the falciparum ligament that is connected near the umbilicus. Along the ventral or anterior surface, the falciparum ligament would occur which tilts itself into the hepatic peritoneal which cover the posterior superiorly so that it can have the left of the anterior portion and right coronary ligaments. Inside the inferior venacava, the center of the ligament with liver and hepatic veins would drain [19]. It was assumed that the falciparum ligament would divide the liver into its two-lobe but it was not holding a true standpoint according to the morphologic anatomy. A round ligament *i.e.*, ligamentum teres is found in the below edge of the falciparum, a part of the obliterated umbilical veins (ductus venous) which connects the umbilical fissure with ligamentum venosum as well as the left branch of the portal veins. In the middle of the lobe of caudate dorsally and the lobe of left ventrally, the ligamentum venosum lies in the fissure which is present at the underlying of the liver area.

During the growth of a baby in a mother's womb, the ductus venosus would carry oxygenated blood to the fetus from the placenta, causing resistance to multiple blood flows of the umbilical veins which is directed towards the superior vena cava. The physiologic neonatal circulation occurs when the baby comes out from the mother's womb in which the closure of the vein relating to the central region of the abdomen (umbilical) has a portal hypertension. The cranial section of the liver is a diaphragmatic surface and there are no ligamentous attachments to the convex areas. Instead, it is connected with the diaphragm through flimsy fibro areolar tissue. The peritoneal reflections of the diaphragm which is responsible for covering the ligament and related to the heart (coronary) is found in the hind and ventral to the base region of liver. This coverage in the left and right parts of the liver will form triangular ligaments to cover both parts of the liver. This helps to fix the position of the liver in the right top quadrant of the abdomen. Through IVC ligament, the control of IVC has a prominent connection with the hepatic lobe which is at the right side, along with the caudate lobe [20]. Meanwhile, Glisson capsule which can be found in the caudate and at the right lobe of the liver is extended to the connection of large membranous tissue. During a surgical operation, the membranous will not only support the organ by keeping it in the position of the liver but it also contains the cells of liver and triads portal. During liver surgery, it also controls unnecessary bleeding or leakage of the bile.

Stomach which is located at the hepatic lobe of the liver and at the left side pass the hepatic ligament of gastro can descend to the side of the omentum which is marginal. It is joined to the tissue which are connected in nature in between the marginal curvature of the stomach and to the lobe which is at the left side and at the ligamentum venosum. The branch hepatic of the vagus nerve end includes neural as well as vascular structure which runs in the gastro-hepatic ligament. The separation of hepatic is found in the diverging of the left liver artery as it originates at the artery which can be found in the left gastric artery. There is a direct reach of the lobe of right hepatic and the portion of the colon which is known as hepatic flexure, a place where the escalated and intersecting colon proceeds to the transverse colon.

The repeat section of liver and other connected biliary and vascular reconstruction are helpful in understanding anatomy. The artery of liver, duct which is common for bile and gall bladder, medial opening vein, posterior and lateral configuration are present in the porta hepatic. In hepatic pancreatic biliary surgery, it is essential to understand the foramen of inflow. This particular inflow was first demonstrated by a Danish anatomist Jacob Winflow in 1732 who had suggested it as a path linking the lesser sac and abdominal cavity. Pringle maneuver [21, 22] which was developed by an Australian physician, James Hogarth Pringle in Glasgow, Scotland would help in the management of the hepatic trauma including the occlusion of the hepatic artery and portal vein inflow by controlling the porta hepatic during the time of hepatic resection which was needed to fully control the hepatic vascular inflow. This procedure can be done by placing a large clamp on the porta-hepatic vein more traumatically by using the tourniquet that passes through the foramen of the Winslow and par flaccid that encircles the porta hepatic. The gallbladder which is placed in the fossa gallbladder at the segments IV and V in the posterior interface connects the common bile ducts *via* the cystic duct. The right hepatic artery branches the cystic artery due to wide varieties of anatomical structure. It is difficult to understand the portal vasculature and biliary anatomy therefore a thorough knowledge is required to avoid any type of injury during the time of hepatic, pancreatic and biliary surgery. On the other hand, the right adrenal gland which is located below the right hepatic lobe can be found in the retroperitoneum. As the right adrenal vein drains into IVC, thorough care is needed while moving the hepatic cell. This is to ensure there will be no vein avulsion or dissection of the adrenal gland that can result in hemorrhage.

Liver drains through shallow and lymphatic network which is supposed to be impenetrable. Furthermore, the production of lymph occurs through the opening vein and it will branchlet the organization which is for drainage of greater lymphatic in the lateral phrenic node by the veins of the liver and the gateway vein's outgrowth [23]. In an anterior and posterior surfaces, the superficial network is placed within the Glisson capsule. The product of drainage of the gateway surface goes into the lymph node which is called phrenic which connects barren region of the liver and the middle and external mammary lymphatic network. The network which is present at the backside would exhaust into the lymph nodes hilar which also include various channels such as cystic channel artery of liver, common bile duct, peripancreatic and lymph nodes celiac. There are surgical implications of the type of lymphatic drainage when it comes to liver, pancreas and gallbladder cancers. Moreover, the control of liver function is quite complicated and the innervation of the neural is yet to be fully comprehended. The liver also has well defined neural innervation. The derived point of nerve fibers is from the celiac plexus lower thoracic ganglia, right phrenic nerve and the vagal from the thorax into the abdomen. The vagus nerves can be divided into two parts *i.e.,* anterior and posterior part. For starters, the anterior part of the vagus nerve is divided into cephalic and hepatic divisions in which the latter one passes along the lesser omentum so that it can facilitate the liver which is needed for the innervation of parasympathetic. From the celiac plexus and thoracic, a splanchnic nerve sympathetic innervation would occur. The liver also is a vascular organ as it receives up to 25% of total cardiac output. It has a dual blood supply which is distinguished equally between the hepatic artery that carries 25% to 30% of blood supply and the portal vein which is required for the remaining 70 to 75%. The two arterial blood and portal will ultimately mix in the sinusoids of the hepatic before it comes out into the circulation throughout the body by the liver venous system [24]. The structures of veins of artery and liver are different. From the celiac axis, the artery which is the common artery of a liver starts in the splenic arteries and at the gastric left side. The artery that comes from the liver will travel sidewise and divide into the gastric duodenal artery and artery of the liver. It provides the pylorus and the duodenum in the proximal position to many indirect divisions into the pancreas. The artery of liver goes in the middle side at the ligament.

The portal vein is responsible for the majority of the liver's nutritional blood supply. Pancreatic portal vessels are formed by the superior mesenteric and splenic vein arising from the pancreatic neck. This vein does not have any valve while the high system of pressure is at the range of 3 – 5 mmHg. As the principal porta systemic shunt during portal hypertension, the left stomach vein, also known as the coronary vein, is clinically significant. In the hepatoduodenal ligament, the main portal vein would penetrate the liver and separate into the left and right portal veins around the hilum. In the liver, the biliary tree is composed of many ducts and it is responsible for the production and transportation of bile, which is then transported to the duodenum by the portal venous system. From segments V and VIII, the duct on the right-side would divide into an anterior sectoral duct and a posterior sectoral duct, which is made up of segments VI and VII. The sectoral duct is located at the anterior, vertically while the posterior duct is situated at the lateral, horizontally. The duct which is on the right side has a short course of extrahepatic branches and there are many branching varieties. The left hepatic duct has fewer varieties and an extended extrahepatic course. Nonetheless, the two duct will be joining near the hilar plate to form a common hepatic duct. Meanwhile, the biliary drain is variable and it can be seen on the right approximately 70 to 80% [25].

To understand the MOA of Liver Toxicity induced by the different class of drugs used in the treatment of acute and chronic diseases *i.e.* Arrhythmia, pain, erectile dysfunction, epilepsy, hypertension and infections, the details are mentioned in Table **1**.

Table 1. MOA of Liver Toxicity by Different Drugs.

Drug Name	Class	Brand Name	Uses	MOA	References
Amiodarone	Class III antiarrhythmic drug	Cordarone	This medication is used to treat extreme irregular heartbeat (ventricular fibrillation)	Cumulative dose causes a type of condition called steatohepatitis.	[26]
Acetaminophen	Analgesic and antipyretic	Tylenol, Calpol, Excedrin	It is used to relieve mild to moderate pain including headache, muscle ache and toothaches	It causes dose-related toxic side effects that lead to hepatocyte injury in the centrilobular region. It causes hepatocyte necrosis.	[27]
Bromofenac	NSAID	Prolensa, Xibrom	It helps in minimizing ocular pain.	It causes encephalopathy, fluid retention.	[28]

Drug Name	Class	Brand Name	Uses	MOA	References
Sildenafil	Phosphodiesterase Inhibitor	Viagra	Used to treat erectile dysfunction	It causes liver hypoxia by which liver damage is minimized through the increase in smooth muscle relaxation which occurs by an increase of the NO level which is generated by sildenafil	[29]
Carbamazepine	Anticonvulsant	Epitol, Tegretol	Used to minimize seizure of epilepsy and it is also taken for nerve pain which is caused by diabetes trigeminal neuralgia.	It caused hepatotoxicity through hypersensitivity reaction.	[30]
Cyclosporin	immunosuppressant	Biocon, Zanetaz	Used for human's organ transplantation by preventing rejection of organs among patients who had undergone surgery.	It causes hepatic metabolism as it interacts with the enzyme cytochrome P450. It decreases the flow of bile which causes hyperbilirubinemia with a high dose.	[31]
Progestin	Oral contraceptive	Alnagest-alnabio	Used to prevent pregnancy	It causes liver enzyme elevation that includes serum aminotransferase elevation by not changing the alkaline phosphatase.	[32]
Methyldopa	$\alpha - 2$ receptor agonists, antihypertensive	Aldomet	Used to prevent high blood pressure	It causes viral hepatitis and immune-mediated toxicity	[33]

(Table 1) cont.....

Drug Name	Class	Brand Name	Uses	MOA	References
Nandrolone	Anabolic steroid	Nandrolone decanoate	Managing anemia caused by kidney disease	It is the cause of the rise of transaminase and acute cholestatic syndrome	[34]
Amoxicillin clavulanate	Penicillin type antibiotic	Augmentin	Inhibiting bacterial growth	The patterns of the liver enzyme are raised and they are generally cholestatic with the rise in alkaline phosphatase and gamma-glutamyl transpeptidase.	[35]

RISK FACTORS

The primary risk factors associated with liver diseases are obesity, diabetes, hypertension, high cholesterol, smoking, alcohol, drug abuse and certain drug interactions.

CLINICAL MENIFESTATIONS

Acute liver disease and liver toxicity are one of the most gradually recognized conditions that may develop into the final stage of liver disease without proper preventive measures and treatment. Till now, a huge spectrum of liver diseases has been reported worldwide, ranging from simple accumulation of fat in the liver to fibrosis, necrosis, cirrhosis, hepatitis, hepatocellular carcinoma, alcohol induced liver disease, non-alcoholic fatty liver disease *etc.*, [36]. Alcoholic liver disease constitutes as the oldest form of liver injury that is known to mankind [37]. On the other hand, non-alcoholic steatohepatitis is the second most etiological factor for liver diseases globally [38]. Alcohol induced liver injury has affected around 10-25% of general population in several countries. It has been found prevailing more in males than females. It also has the potential to progress slowly into steatohepatitis, cirrhosis and liver failure [39]. As the most prevailing liver disease worldwide, non-alcoholic fatty liver disease may lead to advanced fibrosis with time along with several adverse outcomes [40]. It can be more complicated with certain risk factors associated such as type 2 (non-insuli--dependent) diabetes mellitus, obesity, hypertension and hyperlipidemia [41]. These metabolic abnormalities should be addressed in early adulthood to curb high risk of progressive liver disease while at the same time adopting a healthy lifestyle [42].

Symptoms

Some of the patients with liver injury do not show any signs or symptoms during diagnosis while most of them have experienced certain discomfort such as jaundice, dark urine color, nausea, vomiting, abdominal pain, loss of appetite, itching, bloody stool, chronic fatigue, pale and tar colored stool, swelling in the neck and ankles, easy bruising, mental confusion *etc.*, [43, 44].

Diagnosis

The clinical study of non-alcoholic fatty liver disease has disclosed certain possibilities of its occurrence. Table **2** shows the standards for clinical diagnosis of non-alcoholic fatty liver disease. When the following items in A co-exists with any of the items in B, then the clinical diagnosis can be made.

Table 2. Criteria standards for clinical diagnosis of non-alcoholic fatty liver disease [45].

A	B
1. No history of alcohol consumption (<140g in men/ <70g in women)	The imaging tests of liver compliments with the diagnostic standards of diffused fatty liver
2. Absence of disease triggers that can increase the rate of developing liver failure (Hepatitis, drug induced, Wilson's disease)	
3. Disease accompanying with certain non-specific conditions such as mild liver pain, dyspepsia, fatigues and hepatomegaly	The histopathology study compliments with the pathological diagnostic standards of fatty liver
4. Constituents of metabolic syndrome such as visceral, blood lipid disorder, hypertension & hyperglycemia	
5. Sudden elevated levels of liver enzymes	

The specific diagnosis of liver disorders involves clinical history and physical examination that must be performed by a physician or healthcare professional to understand the root of injury and suggest the necessary diagnostic tests such as Gamma-glutamyl transferase (GGT), Serum glutamic pyruvic transaminase (SGPT)/ Serum glutamic oxaloacetic transaminase(SGOT), alkaline phosphatase, bilirubin tests, proteins & albumin test, liver biopsy *etc.*, afterwards [46, 47]. The diagnosis of liver injury or liver toxicity depends upon a series of features that includes patient's history of significant intake of alcohol, smoking habits, drug induced toxicity *etc.* However, this process will pose some difficulties to diagnose the disease particularly when patients would refrain from providing correct information regarding alcohol abuse [48]. As for the physical examination, the evaluation often requires examining the entire body to reveal the severity of the disease. Liver biopsy is the most appropriate and tactful method to detect fatty liver disease as it can still produce sufficient results (alcoholic or non-alcoholic) even though it cannot provide reliable distinction for the cause of the disease [49, 50]. Biopsy is suggested only when the etiology is not clear and the confirmatory for the stage of disease is needed be recognized. Liver tissue samples obtained from the biopsy can be utilized to approach the topographical spread of fibrosis by making use of several staining techniques, which in turn offer the possibility to carry out molecular studies [51]. There are other diagnostic tests include ultrasound CT scan and fibro scan [52]. Hepatomegaly is the most frequent condition found in majority of the patients [53]. For children with non-alcoholic liver disease, Acanthosis nigricans may be common [54]. Some patients with non-alcoholic fatty liver disease show very less or no symptoms at the time of diagnosis while some would report feeling of discomfort and malaise on the right upper abdominal region. In an advanced liver disease, which is approaching to cirrhosis, disruption of hepatic biosynthesis can occur and may lead to thrombocytopenia.

For diseases like liver cirrhosis, the diagnosis is done through ultrasonography techniques which reflects non-uniform hepatic tissue, asymmetrical surfaces of hepatic region, caudate lobe enlargement, portal hypertension which can eventually lead to splenomegaly. There are no well-established and defined threshold values for laboratory tests which can be referred to while confirming cirrhosis [55]. Supplementary studies include gastroscopy and ultrasonography, Esophagogastroduodenoscopy (EGD) can be useful to detect varices present in esophageal region. However, non-invasive techniques are only utilized when the physician wants to diagnose the stage of fibrosis rather than the physiological condition of the liver. Not only that, the hepatic diseases also can be diagnosed by analyzing the serum concentrations of a variety of serum analytes. The abnormalities obtained will be correlated with the type of liver disease [56].

Etiology

There have been contradicting reports in which western countries have suggested that the main cause of the final stage of liver disease is hepatitis C virus infection while a group of scientists in Mexico have reported alcohol to be the main cause of liver cirrhosis [57]. Currently, the second leading cause of liver disorders in adults is non-alcoholic steatohepatitis. The etiology behind alcoholic liver disease is not completely understood but it is believed to be due to the toxic effects of alcohol and its intermediate, acetaldehyde [58]. Non-alcoholic fatty liver disease (NAFLD) is closely related to obesity and type 2 diabetes which can further complicate the disease and progress rapidly towards more advanced phase [59]. The mechanisms that regulate hepatic accumulation of lipid and the susceptibility to tissue fibrosis and inflammation are still not fully understood but they provide an indication of a complex relationship between metabolic target tissues which include skeletal muscle, adipose tissues, immune cells and inflammatory cells [59]. Weight loss is one of the major aspects found among patients undergoing treatment for liver disfunction [60]. When it comes to hepatocellular carcinoma, the primary risk factors are diabetes, obesity, high calorie intake, high alcohol intake, chronic infection from hepatitis B and hepatitis C virus and inherited diseases. These factors are also facilitated with a sedentary lifestyle [61]. With the increase in screening, vaccines and anti-viral treatments, the possible burden of chronic liver diseases has been reduced but trigger factors such as drug and alcohol abuse as well as other metabolic syndromes can endanger the trend [62]. Additionally, the progression of liver disease can slowly lead to malnutrition thus, they should be identified in the early stage of diagnosis to correct any recognizable nutrition deficit. This may be due to the incapability of liver to store essential nutrients, malabsorption and metabolic disturbances [63]. Weight loss is another important risk factor associated with liver cirrhosis but the etiology behind it is yet to be thoroughly investigated. Patients would experience significant weight loss in alcoholic cirrhosis as compared to hepatitis C virus and autoimmune hepatitis [60].

Liver transplantation is the ultimate and definitive treatment option for patients who are at the final stage of liver disease [64]. Despite huge clinical trial for decades, there is no single treatment strategy suggested for non-alcoholic fatty liver disease [65]. However, a number of treatment options are already available to treat hepatocellular carcinoma including local ablation, surgical resection, radiofrequency, radioembolization, transcatheter arterial chemoembolization (TACE) and systemic targeted candidates like sorafenib, depending on the stage of liver and associated liver dysfunction [66]. Some PPARG agonists and metformin have been found to improve prognosis and lower the risk of hepatocellular carcinoma [67].

FUTURE PROSPECTS

With the recent advancement in science, various diagnostic techniques are available to solve the crises associated with early detection of liver disease. Presently, the available drugs have met the market demand. However, prevention should include in the form of awareness relating to the risk factors associated with liver disease to better manage the disease in future. Early diagnosis or detection of liver disease will help patients to avoid complicated surgeries and expensive medicines. Drug induced hepatoxicity also should be checked as the side effects associated in most of the drugs is liver toxicity.

CONCLUSION

In this chapter, we have covered the vast knowledge of the different aspects of liver *i.e.*, anatomy, physiology, pathophysiology and related advancement to overcome the problems of liver diseases and also focused on how to maintain a healthy liver. This chapter will play an important role in the area of medical science and will be used as a reference tool for the medical team, scientist, researcher and society which definitely will decrease the rate of hepatotoxicity in the world population.

REFERENCES

[1]   Bismuth, H. Surgical anatomy and anatomical surgery of the liver. *World J. Surg.,* **1982**, *6*(1), 3-9.
       [http://dx.doi.org/10.1007/BF01656368] [PMID: 7090393]

[2]   Baskaran, V.; Banerjee, J.K.; Ghosh, S.R.; Kumar, S.S.; Anand, S.; Menon, G.; Mishra, D.S.; Saranga Bharathi, R. Applications of hepatic round ligament/falciform ligament flap and graft in abdominal surgery : A review of their utility and efficacy. *Langenbecks Arch. Surg.,* **2021**, *406*(5), 1249-1281.
       [http://dx.doi.org/10.1007/s00423-020-02031-6] [PMID: 33411036]

[3]   Stanger, B.Z.; Tanaka, A.J.; Melton, D.A. Organ size is limited by the number of embryonic progenitor cells in the pancreas but not the liver. *Nature,* **2007**, *445*(7130), 886-891.
       [http://dx.doi.org/10.1038/nature05537] [PMID: 17259975]

[4]   Shipley, L.A.; Davila, T.B.; Thines, N.J.; Elias, B.A. Nutritional requirements and diet choices of the pygmy rabbit (*Brachylagus idahoensis*): A sagebrush specialist. *J. Chem. Ecol.,* **2006**, *32*(11), 2455-2474.
       [http://dx.doi.org/10.1007/s10886-006-9156-2] [PMID: 17082988]

[5]   Protzer, U.; Maini, M.K.; Knolle, P.A. Living in the liver: Hepatic infections. *Nat. Rev. Immunol.,* **2012**, *12*(3), 201-213.
       [http://dx.doi.org/10.1038/nri3169] [PMID: 22362353]

[6]   Wojciechowski, V.V.; Calina, D.; Tsarouhas, K.; Pivnik, A.V.; Sergievich, A.A.; Kodintsev, V.V.; Filatova, E.A.; Ozcagli, E.; Docea, A.O.; Arsene, A.L.; Gofita, E.; Tsitsimpikou, C.; Tsatsakis, A.M.; Golokhvast, K.S. A guide to acquired vitamin K coagulophathy diagnosis and treatment: The Russian perspective. *Daru,* **2017**, *25*(1), 10.
       [http://dx.doi.org/10.1186/s40199-017-0175-z] [PMID: 28416008]

[7]   Kullak-Ublick, G.A.; Andrade, R.J.; Merz, M.; End, P.; Benesic, A.; Gerbes, A.L.; Aithal, G.P. Drug-induced liver injury: Recent advances in diagnosis and risk assessment. *Gut,* **2017**, *66*(6), 1154-1164.
       [http://dx.doi.org/10.1136/gutjnl-2016-313369] [PMID: 28341748]

[8]   Vuppalanchi, R.; Liangpunsakul, S.; Chalasani, N. Etiology of new-onset jaundice: how often is it caused by idiosyncratic drug-induced liver injury in the united states? *Am. J. Gastroenterol.,* **2007**, *102*(3), 558-562.
       [http://dx.doi.org/10.1111/j.1572-0241.2006.01019.x] [PMID: 17156142]

[9]   Reuben, A.; Koch, D.G.; Lee, W.M. Drug-induced acute liver failure: Results of a U.S. multicenter, prospective study. *Hepatology,* **2010**, *52*(6), 2065-2076.
       [http://dx.doi.org/10.1002/hep.23937] [PMID: 20949552]

[10]   Zimmerman, H.J. Hepatotoxicity: The adverse effects of drugs and other chemicals on the liver. Lippincott Williams & Wilkins: Philadelphia, **1999**.

[11]   LiverTox: clinical and research information on drug-induced liver injury. Bethesda, MD: National Institutes of Health https://www.LiverTox.nih.gov

[12] Larson, A.M.; Polson, J.; Fontana, R.J.; Davern, T.J.; Lalani, E.; Hynan, L.S.; Reisch, J.S.; Schiødt, F.V.; Ostapowicz, G.; Shakil, A.O.; Lee, W.M. Acetaminophen-induced acute liver failure: Results of a United States multicenter, prospective study. *Hepatology,* **2005**, *42*(6), 1364-1372. [http://dx.doi.org/10.1002/hep.20948] [PMID: 16317692]

[13] Dalton, T.A.; Berry, R.S. Hepatotoxicity associated with sustained-release niacin. *Am. J. Med.,* **1992**, *93*(1), 102-104. [http://dx.doi.org/10.1016/0002-9343(92)90689-9] [PMID: 1626557]

[14] Björnsson, E.S.; Bergmann, O.M.; Björnsson, H.K.; Kvaran, R.B.; Olafsson, S. Incidence, presentation, and outcomes in patients with drug-induced liver injury in the general population of Iceland. *Gastroenterology,* **2013**, *144*(7), 1419-1425.e3. [http://dx.doi.org/10.1053/j.gastro.2013.02.006] [PMID: 23419359]

[15] Chalasani, N.; Bonkovsky, H.L.; Fontana, R.; Lee, W.; Stolz, A.; Talwalkar, J.; Reddy, K.R.; Watkins, P.B.; Navarro, V.; Barnhart, H.; Gu, J.; Serrano, J. Features and outcomes of 889 patients with drug-induced liver injury: The DILIN Prospective Study. *Gastroenterology,* **2015**, *148*(7), 1340-52.e7. [http://dx.doi.org/10.1053/j.gastro.2015.03.006] [PMID: 25754159]

[16] Sgro, C.; Clinard, F.; Ouazir, K.; Chanay, H.; Allard, C.; Guilleminet, C.; Lenoir, C.; Lemoine, A.; Hillon, P. Incidence of drug-induced hepatic injuries: A french population-based study. *Hepatology,* **2002**, *36*(2), 451-455. [http://dx.doi.org/10.1053/jhep.2002.34857] [PMID: 12143055]

[17] Captur, G.; Karperien, A.L.; Hughes, A.D.; Francis, D.P.; Moon, J.C. The fractal heart :Embracing mathematics in the cardiology clinic. *Nat. Rev. Cardiol.,* **2017**, *14*(1), 56-64. [http://dx.doi.org/10.1038/nrcardio.2016.161] [PMID: 27708281]

[18] Yoshino K, Taura K, Takaori K, Kasai Y, Hatano E. Surgical anatomy of the liver. Surgical Anatomy of the Liver. In:, et al. The IASGO Textbook of Multi-Disciplinary Management of Hepato-Pancreat--Biliary Diseases. Springer, Singapore. 2022; 1-6. [http://dx.doi.org/10.1007/978-981-19-0063-1_1]

[19] Jamieson, G.G. The anatomy of general surgical operations. Churchill Livingstone/Elsevier: Edinburgh, NY, **2006**; pp. 8-23.

[20] Kogure, K.; Ishizaki, M.; Nemoto, M.; Kuwano, H.; Yorifuji, H.; Ishikawa, H.; Takata, K.; Makuuchi, M. Close relation between the inferior vena cava ligament and the caudate lobe in the human liver. *J. Hepatobiliary Pancreat. Surg.,* **2007**, *14*(3), 297-301. [http://dx.doi.org/10.1007/s00534-006-1148-7] [PMID: 17520206]

[21] Pringle, J.H. Notes on the arrest of hepatic hemorrhage due to trauma. *Ann. Surg.,* **1908**, *48*(4), 541-549. [http://dx.doi.org/10.1097/00000658-190810000-00005] [PMID: 17862242]

[22] van Gulik, T.M.; de Graaf, W.; Dinant, S.; Busch, O.R.C.; Gouma, D.J. Vascular occlusion techniques during liver resection. *Dig. Surg.,* **2007**, *24*(4), 274-281. [http://dx.doi.org/10.1159/000103658] [PMID: 17657152]

[23] Skandalakis, J.E.; Skandalakis, L.J.; Skandalakis, P.N.; Mirilas, P. Hepatic surgical anatomy. *Surg. Clin. North Am.,* **2004**, *84*(2), 413-435, viii. [http://dx.doi.org/10.1016/j.suc.2003.12.002] [PMID: 15062653]

[24] Blumgart, L.H.; Belghiti, J. Surgery of the liver, biliary tract, and pancreas. Saunders Elsevier: Philadelphia, **2007**; pp. 3-30. [http://dx.doi.org/10.1016/B978-1-4160-3256-4.50009-0]

[25] Sherif, R.Z.; Abdel-Misih, Mark Bloomston Liver anatomy. *Surg. Clin. North Am.,* **2010**, *90*(4), 643-653. [http://dx.doi.org/10.1016/j.suc.2010.04.017] [PMID: 20637938]

[26] Yong, R.; Zhiqi, K.; Chan, L.; Shiyao, G.; Yaohao, X.; Dandan, Z.; Yutao, H.; Bingbing, S.; Zhi, J.;

Zhenhuang, G.; Xiyuan, L.; Chengdao, L.; Shuobin, C.; Jiming, Y.; Zhishu, H.; Yongjun, L. Gut Akkermansiamuciniphila ameliorates metabolic dysfunction-associated fatty liver disease by regulating the metabolism of L-aspartate *via* gut-liver axis. *Gut Microbes,* **2021**, *13*, 1.

[27]   Jendrzejewska, I.; Goryczka, T.; Pietrasik, E.; Klimontko, J.; Jampilek, J. X-ray and thermal analysis of selected drugs containing acetaminophen. *Molecules,* **2020**, *25*(24), 5909.
[http://dx.doi.org/10.3390/molecules25245909] [PMID: 33322235]

[28]   Coassin, M.; De Maria, M.; Mastrofilippo, V.; Braglia, L.; Cimino, L.; Sartori, A.; Fontana, L. Anterior chamber inflammation after cataract surgery: A randomized clinical trial comparing bromfenac 0.09% to dexamethasone 0.1%. *Adv. Ther.,* **2019**, *36*(10), 2712-2722.
[http://dx.doi.org/10.1007/s12325-019-01076-4] [PMID: 31482510]

[29]   Bermejo, J.; Yotti, R.; García-Orta, R.; Sánchez-Fernández, P.L.; Castaño, M.; Segovia-Cubero, J.; Escribano-Subías, P.; San Román, J.A.; Borrás, X.; Alonso-Gómez, A.; Botas, J.; Crespo-Leiro, M.G.; Velasco, S.; Bayés-Genís, A.; López, A.; Muñoz-Aguilera, R.; de Teresa, E.; González-Juanatey, J.R.; Evangelista, A.; Mombiela, T.; González-Mansilla, A.; Elízaga, J.; Martín-Moreiras, J.; González-Santos, J.M.; Moreno-Escobar, E.; Fernández-Avilés, F.; Bermejo, J.; Yotti, R.; Mombiela, T.; Gónzález-Mansilla, A.; Elízaga, J.; García-Robles, J.A.; Pérez-David, E.; Pérez del Villar, C.; Sanz, R.; Guticrrcz-Ibanes, E.; Vázquez, M.E.; Mur, A.; Benito, Y.; Martínez-Legazpi, P.; Barrio, A.; Vázquez, A.; García-Orta, R.; Uribe, I.; González, M.; Luis Sánchez, P.; González-Santos, J.M.; Martín-Moreiras, J.; Arribas, A.; Clemente Lorenzo, M.M.; Diego Nieto, A.; Castaño, M.; Pérez de Prado, A.; Alonso, D.; Segovia-Cubero, J.; Gómez-Bueno, M.; Sayago Silva, I.; Ángel Cavero, M.; Escribano-Subias, P.; Domínguez, L.; Tello de Meneses, R.; Ruiz Cano, M.J.; Jiménez López-Guarch, C.; San Román, J.A.; Mota, P.; Borrás, X.; Amorós Galitó, C.; Alonso-Gómez, A.; Belló Mora, M.C.; Mesa Rubio, D.; Botas, J.; Campuzano, R.; Crespo-Leiro, M.G.; Marzoa, R.; Cuenca, J.; Velasco, S.; Muñoz, R.; Suberviola, V.; Beltrán Herrera, C.; Mora, L.; Mar Sarrión, M.; Vaqueriza, D.; Bayes-Genís, A.; Ferrer, E.; González-Juanatey, J.R.; Cid, B.; Monzonís, A.M.; López, A.; Arizón de Prado, J.M.; Santisteban, M.; Mesa Rubio, D.; Evangelista, A.; García-Dorado, D.; de Teresa, E.; Jiménez-Navarro, M.; Carrasco Chinchilla, F.; Moreno-Escobar, E.; Alonso, J. Sildenafil for improving outcomes in patients with corrected valvular heart disease and persistent pulmonary hypertension: A multicenter, double-blind, randomized clinical trial. *Eur. Heart J.,* **2018**, *39*(15), 1255-1264.
[http://dx.doi.org/10.1093/eurheartj/ehx700]

[30]   Janković, S.M. Evaluation of zonisamide for the treatment of focal epilepsy: A review of pharmacokinetics, clinical efficacy and adverse effects. *Expert Opin. Drug Metab. Toxicol.,* **2020**, *16*(3), 169-177.
[http://dx.doi.org/10.1080/17425255.2020.1736035] [PMID: 32116059]

[31]   Sanchez-Pernaute O, Romero-Bueno FI, Selva-O'Callaghan A. Why Choose Cyclosporin A as First-line Therapy in COVID-19 Pneumonia [published online ahead of print. 16 Reumatol Clin (Engl Ed). 2020;S1699-258X(20)30044-9.

[32]   Flores, V.A.; Vanhie, A.; Dang, T.; Taylor, H.S. Progesterone receptor status predicts response to progestin therapy in endometriosis. *J. Clin. Endocrinol. Metab.,* **2018**, *103*(12), 4561-4568.
[http://dx.doi.org/10.1210/jc.2018-01227] [PMID: 30357380]

[33]   Tajik, S.; Beitollahi, H.; Biparva, P. Methyldopa electrochemical sensor based on a glassy carbon electrode modified with Cu/TiO2 nanocomposite. *J. Serb. Chem. Soc.,* **2018**, *83*(7-8), 863-874.
[http://dx.doi.org/10.2298/JSC170930024T]

[34]   Patanè, F.G.; Liberto, A.; Maria Maglitto, A.N.; Malandrino, P.; Esposito, M.; Amico, F.; Cocimano, G.; Rosi, G.L.; Condorelli, D.; Nunno, N.D.; Montana, A. Nandrolone decanoate: use, abuse and side effects. *Medicina,* **2020**, *56*(11), 606.
[http://dx.doi.org/10.3390/medicina56110606] [PMID: 33187340]

[35]   Veeraraghavan, B.; Bakthavatchalam, Y.D.; Sahni, R.D. Orally administered amoxicillin/clavulanate: Current role in outpatient therapy. *Infect. Dis. Ther.,* **2021**, *10*(1), 15-25.
[http://dx.doi.org/10.1007/s40121-020-00374-7] [PMID: 33306184]

[36]   Satapathy, SK; Sanyal, AJ Epidemiology and natural history of nonalcoholic fatty liver disease. *Semin Liver Dis.,* **2015**, *35*(3), 221-235.
[http://dx.doi.org/10.1055/s-0035-1562943]

[37]   Shea, RSO; Dasarathy, S; Mccullough, AJ; Committee, G Practice Guideline committee of the american association for the study of liver diseases; practice parameters committee of the american college of gastroenterology. *Alcoholic liver disease. Hepatology.,* **2010**, 51(1), 307-328.
[http://dx.doi.org/10.1002/hep.23258]

[38]   Chalasani, N The diagnosis and management of non-alcoholic fatty liver disease: practice guideline by the american association for the study of liver diseases, american college of gastroenterology, and the american gastroenterological association. *Hepatology,* **2012**, *55*(6), 2005-2023.
[http://dx.doi.org/10.1002/hep.25762]

[39]   Ct, L Hepatic steatosis *(fatty liver disease*) in asymptomatic adults identified by unenhanced low-dose CT. *AJR Am J Roentgenol.,* **2010**, *194*(3), 623-628.
[http://dx.doi.org/10.2214/AJR.09.2590]

[40]   Rinella, M. NAFLD 2020 : The state of the disease correspondence. *Gastroenterology,* **2020**, *158*(7), 1851-1864.
[http://dx.doi.org/10.1053/j.gastro.2020.01.052]

[41]   Angulo, P. Nonalcoholic fatty liver disease. *N. Engl. J. Med.,* **2002**, *346*(16), 1221-1231.
[http://dx.doi.org/10.1056/NEJMra011775] [PMID: 11961152]

[42]   Younossi, ZM; Marchesini, G; Pinto-cortez, H; Petta, S epidemiology of nonalcoholic fatty liver disease and nonalcoholic steatohepatitis: Implications for liver transplantation. *Transplantation.,* **2019**, *103*(1), 22-27.

[43]   Newton, J.L. Systemic symptoms in non-alcoholic fatty liver disease. *Dig. Dis.,* **2010**, *28*(1), 214-219.
[http://dx.doi.org/10.1159/000282089] [PMID: 20460914]

[44]   Kobelska-Dubiel, N.; Klincewicz, B.; Cichy, W. Liver disease in cystic fibrosis. *Prz. Gastroenterol.,* **2014**, *3*(3), 136-141.
[http://dx.doi.org/10.5114/pg.2014.43574] [PMID: 25097709]

[45]   Zeng, MD; Fan, JG; Lu, LG; Li, YM; Chen, CW; Wang, BY; Mao, BY Chinese National Consensus Workshop on Nonalcoholic Fatty Liver Disease. Guidelines for the diagnosis and treatment of nonalcoholic fatty liver diseases. *J Dig Dis.,* **2008**, *9*(2), 108-112.
[http://dx.doi.org/10.1111/j.1751-2980.2008.00331.x]

[46]   Dyson, J.K.; Anstee, Q.M.; McPherson, S. Non-alcoholic fatty liver disease: A practical approach to diagnosis and staging. *Frontline Gastroenterol.,* **2014**, *5*(3), 211-218.
[http://dx.doi.org/10.1136/flgastro-2013-100403] [PMID: 25018867]

[47]   Torruellas, C.; French, S.W.; Medici, V. Diagnosis of alcoholic liver disease. *World J. Gastroenterol.,* **2014**, *20*(33), 11684-11699.
[http://dx.doi.org/10.3748/wjg.v20.i33.11684] [PMID: 25206273]

[48]   Ahmed, Z.; Ahmed, U.; Walayat, S.; Ren, J.; Martin, D.K.; Moole, H.; Koppe, S.; Yong, S.; Dhillon, S. Liver function tests in identifying patients with liver disease. *Clin. Exp. Gastroenterol.,* **2018**, *11*, 301-307.
[http://dx.doi.org/10.2147/CEG.S160537] [PMID: 30197529]

[49]   Clark, JM; Brancati, FL; Diehl, AMAE Nonalcoholic fatty liver disease. *Gastroenterology.,* **2002**, *122*(6), 1649-1657.
[http://dx.doi.org/10.1053/gast.2002.33573]

[50]   Choudhury, J; Sanyal, AJ Clinical aspects of fatty liver disease. *Semin Liver Dis.,* **2004**, *24*(4), 349-362.
[http://dx.doi.org/10.1055/s-2004-860864]

[51]   Pinzani, M; Rombouts, K; Colagrande, S. Fibrosis in chronic liver diseases: Diagnosis and management. *J Hepatol.,* **2005**, *42*1, S22-S36.
[http://dx.doi.org/10.1016/j.jhep.2004.12.008]

[52]   Carey, E.; Carey, W.D. Noninvasive tests for liver disease, fibrosis, and cirrhosis: Is liver biopsy obsolete? *Cleve. Clin. J. Med.,* **2010**, *77*(8), 519-527.
[http://dx.doi.org/10.3949/ccjm.77a.09138] [PMID: 20682514]

[53]   Roberts, E.A. Non-alcoholic steatohepatitis in children. *Clin. Liver Dis.,* **2007**, *11*(1), 155-172, x.
[http://dx.doi.org/10.1016/j.cld.2007.02.008] [PMID: 17544977]

[54]   Manton, N.D.; Lipsett, J.; Moore, D.J.; Davidson, G.P.; Bourne, A.J.; Couper, R.T.L. Non-alcoholic steatohepatitis in children and adolescents. *Med. J. Aust.,* **2000**, *173*(9), 476-479.
[http://dx.doi.org/10.5694/j.1326-5377.2000.tb139299.x] [PMID: 11149304]

[55]   Wiegand, J.; Berg, T. The etiology, diagnosis and prevention of liver cirrhosis: Part 1 of a series on liver cirrhosis. *Dtsch Arztebl Int.,* **2013**, *110*(6), 85-89.

[56]   Wolf, P.L. Biochemical Diagnosis of Liver Disease. *Indian Journal of Clinical Biochemistry,* **1999**, *14*, 59-90.

[57]   Méndez-sánchez, N; Aguilar-ramírez, JR; Reyes, A; Dehesa, M Etiology of liver cirrhosis in mexico. *Annals of Hepatology,* **2004**, *3*(1), 30-33.
[http://dx.doi.org/10.1016/S1665-2681(19)32122-2]

[58]   Stickel, F.; Datz, C.; Hampe, J.; Bataller, R. Pathophysiology and management of alcoholic liver disease: Update 2016. *Gut Liver,* **2017**, *11*(2), 173-188.
[http://dx.doi.org/10.5009/gnl16477] [PMID: 28274107]

[59]   Marjot, T.; Moolla, A.; Cobbold, J.F.; Hodson, L.; Tomlinson, J.W. Nonalcoholic fatty liver disease in adults: Current concepts in etiology, outcomes, and management. *Endocr. Rev.,* **2020**, *41*(1), 66-117.
[http://dx.doi.org/10.1210/endrev/bnz009] [PMID: 31629366]

[60]   Anastácio; Lucilene Rezende; Lívia Garcia Ferreira; Hélem de Sena Ribeiro; Agnaldo Soares Lima; Eduardo Garcia Vilela; and Maria Isabel Toulson Davisson Correia. Weight loss during cirrhosis is related to the etiology of liver disease. Arquivos de gastroenterologia **2012**, 195-198.

[61]   Yang, J.D.; Hainaut, P.; Gores, G.J.; Amadou, A.; Plymoth, A.; Roberts, L.R. A global view of hepatocellular carcinoma: Trends, risk, prevention and management. *Nat. Rev. Gastroenterol. Hepatol.,* **2019**, *16*(10), 589-604.
[http://dx.doi.org/10.1038/s41575-019-0186-y] [PMID: 31439937]

[62]   Moon, AM; Singal, AG; Tapper, EB Contemporary epidemiology of chronic liver disease and cirrhosis. *Clin Gastroenterol Hepatol.,* **2019**, *18*(12), 2650-2666.
[http://dx.doi.org/10.1016/j.cgh.2019.07.060]

[63]   Johnson, T.M.; Overgard, E.B.; Cohen, A.E.; Dibaise, J.K. Nutrition assessment and management in advanced liver disease. *Nutr. Clin. Pract.,* **2014**, 14-29.
[http://dx.doi.org/10.1177/0884533612469027] [PMID: 23319353]

[64]   Singal, A.K. Evolving frequency and outcomes of liver transplantation based on etiology of liver disease. *Transplantation,* **2013**, *95*, 755-760.

[65]   Ahmed, A.; Wong, R.J.; Harrison, S.A. NAFLD review: Diagnosis, treatment and outcomes. *Clin. Gastroenterol. Hepatol.,* **2015**, *13*(12), 2062-2070.
[http://dx.doi.org/10.1016/j.cgh.2015.07.029] [PMID: 26226097]

[66]   Suresh, D.; Srinivas, A.N.; Kumar, D.P. Etiology of hepatocellular carcinoma: Special focus on fatty liver disease. *Front. Oncol.,* **2020**, *10*, 601710.
[http://dx.doi.org/10.3389/fonc.2020.601710] [PMID: 33330100]

[67]   Baffy, G; Brunt, EM; Caldwell, SH Hepatocellular carcinoma in non-alcoholic fatty liver disease: An emerging menace. *J Hepatol.,* **2012**, *56*(6), 1384-1391.

CHAPTER 2

Hepatoprotective Role of Medicinal Plants

Bedanta Bhattacharjee[1]**, Tirna Paul**[1]**, Retno Widyowati**[2]**, Ram Kumar Sahu**[3,*] **and Monika Kaurav**[4]

[1] *Department of Pharmaceutical Sciences, Faculty of Science and Engineering, Dibrugarh University, Dibrugarh-786004, Assam, India*

[2] *Department of Pharmaceutical Science, Faculty of Pharmacy, Universitas Airlangga, Surabaya, 60115, Indonesia*

[3] *Department of Pharmaceutical Sciences, Hemvati Nandan Bahuguna Garhwal University (A Central University), Chauras Campus, Tehri Garhwal-249161, Uttarakhand, India*

[4] *KIET School of Pharmacy, KIET Groups of Institutions, Delhi-NCR, Meerut Road (NH-58) Ghaziabad – 201206, India*

Abstract: With its ability to self-regenerate, the liver is considered an important gland in the human body, performing essential functions such as the production of vital proteins, lipids, lipoproteins, glucose homeostasis as well as the production and secretion of vitamin stores and bile acids. Therefore, any impairment of the organ can lead to serious problems in our bodies. There are various forms of disorders associated with an unhealthy liver, which affect the liver in different ways and can be detected by observing various general symptoms and some specific diagnostic tests. To treat and control these hazardous effects on our bodies, various medicines are available in the market that are mainly derived from plants and plant products. As they have fewer side effects, herbal medicines have attracted much attention for alleviating various liver diseases while maintaining a healthy lifestyle. Moreover, nanobased delivery of natural products shows higher hepatoprotective activity than crude extracts. In this chapter, various hepatoprotective functions of medicinal plants and their nano-based drug delivery have been highlighted.

Keywords: Liver, Homeostasis, Lipoprotein, Disorders, Tests, Herbal drugs, Mitigation.

INTRODUCTION

The liver is an important gland in the human body. Due to its essential role in the human body, our entire body function will be affected if our liver is impaired. The liver also has the ability to regenerate itself. It serves to provide biological mole-

---

* **Corresponding author Ram Kumar Sahu:** Department of Pharmaceutical Sciences, Hemvati Nandan Bahuguna Garhwal University (A Central University), Chauras Campus, Tehri Garhwal-249161, Uttarakhand, India; Email: ramsahu79@gmail.com

Sachin Kumar Jain, Ram Kumar Sahu, Priyanka Soni, Vishal Soni & Shiv Shankar Shukla (Eds.)

-cules and detoxify toxins. The essential functions of the liver include the production of vital proteins, lipids and lipoproteins, glucose homeostasis as well as the production and secretion of vitamin stores and bile acids [1]. Any damage to the liver can lead to severe consequences [2]. These include fibrosis, cell necrosis, decreased tissue glutathione levels and increased tissue lipid peroxidation. Furthermore, toxic chemicals, drugs, foods and infections, such as parasites, viruses, bacteria and fungi can lead to various liver dysfunctions or diseases such as jaundice, liver cancer, hepatitis and cirrhosis.

The liver also plays a central role in the production and secretion of bile juice which is used for the breakdown and digestion of fatty acids. It produces blood clotting factors *i.e.* prothrombin and fibrinogen. It also produces mucopolysaccharide sulphuric acid ester *i.e.* heparin, which prevents blood clotting in the blood vessels of the circulatory system. In the digestive system, it generates hundreds of enzymes and blood proteins for various bodily functions. Apart from that, the liver also produces urea, breaks down proteins, stores trace elements including copper, and iron along with vitamins A, B12, and D, and helps to neutralise drugs and toxins. It also filters our blood and eliminates harmful substances from the blood. Moreover, it helps in the elimination of excess hormones, and managing blood sugar by maintaining the optimal blood sugar level. The poorly functioning liver can lead to hypoglycaemia or diabetes. Besides, an impaired liver can cause an inability to fight infections as our liver has the ability to eliminate certain bacterial and general infections.

Maintaining a healthy liver is important to secure a healthy life. However, an unhealthy lifestyle and various other reasons can lead to liver dysfunction. There are various signs and symptoms which can help in the early detection of liver diseases or its dysfunction such as dark urine, discoloration, yellowish eyes, nail and skin, yellow, gray or pale stool, vomiting with or without blood, nausea, black or bloody stools, loss of appetite, unusually prolonged itching, weight fluctuation, mental confusion, sleep disturbance, abdominal pain, loss of stamina, fatigue and many more. There are other symptoms that may be experienced due to autointoxication thus indicating that our liver must be cleaned. This is a process in which our body, through improper digestion, elimination, *etc.*, has poisoned the substances it produces on its own. These signs and symptoms include hair breakage, acne outbreaks, insomnia or bad dreams, flu-like feelings, exhaustion, an imbalance in blood sugar levels, and difficulty concentrating and thinking.

The most common liver diseases include hepatitis, jaundice, liver cancer and cirrhosis. Hepatitis is usually caused by viruses and it refers to the inflammation of the liver. Other reasons include chemicals, alcohol or other autoimmune hypersensitivity reactions. The most common hepatitis viruses are hepatitis A, B, C, D and E [3]. Jaundice, on the other hand, is the result of abnormal metabolism and retention of bilirubin. An early sign of jaundice is when our skin, nails, and eyes have turned yellowish which indicates over circulation of bile. Jaundice can also cause itching on the body [3]. Cirrhosis is a chronic degenerative liver disease in which the parenchymal tissue degenerates while the lobules are interspersed with fats which leads to the formation of perilobular connective tissue. Severe cirrhosis can lead to hepatic coma, ammonia poisoning, renal failure or gastrointestinal bleeding [3].

Even in ancient times, plants played a central role in healthy living. In developing countries, herbal medicines have great importance to people. For the treatment of liver diseases, various herbal drugs have been studied and shown hepatoprotective effects and can be considered hepatoprotective agents. With that, various chemical constituents have been isolated which are responsible for the hepatoprotective effect [4].

For the treatment of liver disorders, a decoction consisting of numerous herbs with multiple properties individually is commonly used. Herbal decoction nourishes our whole body and focuses on treating the liver [5 - 7]. Herbal plants showing hepatoprotective nature include *Andographis paniculata, Embelia ribes, Zingiber officinale, Picrorhiza kurroa, Terminalia chebula, Cichorium intybus, Emblica officinalis (*amla fruit), *Terminalia arjuna, Berberis vulgaris, Phyllanthus niruri, Lawsonia inermis* (henna), and *Aloe barbadensis etc.*

The treatment of liver disorders in allopathic medicines is limited. Furthermore, allopathic drugs such as interferon and corticosteroids are too expensive and have a high risk of side effects and adverse effects [8]. Moreover, their efficacy and effectiveness are limited. Herbal medicines, on the other hand, are inexpensive and easily accessible. They are harmless substitutes for allopathic medicines as they occur naturally and are gentle. Over time, surveys have shown that 65% of hepatic patients have started taking herbal preparations.

Significance of Medicinal Plants in the Management of Liver Toxicity

Liver disorders are very common nowadays. There are various possible causes of liver toxicity. There are also medicines for various liver problems such as allopathic medicines and herbal medicines. Allopathic medicines may show adverse effects and they can be considered too expensive. They have limited effectiveness while herbal medicines are safe, and gentle and do not cause adverse effects. They are cost-effective in the long term. In Ayurveda, herbal substances are used to protect against liver damage by using various dietary agents and chemicals. Therefore, herbal medicines are considered safe and have the potential to cure liver diseases. Due to this, they have gained great popularity of late. Medicinal plants that have the potential to cure liver diseases are considered hepatoprotective drugs. The popularity of medicinal plants over Western medicines is increasing day by day. About 160 phytochemicals and phytoconstituents have been reported to have hepatoprotective activity [9]. In India, over 87 plants have been used out of which 37 are patented and have their own plant formulation consisting of several constituents [10].

APPLICATION OF MEDICINAL PLANTS IN THE MANAGEMENT OF LIVER DISEASE

The use of plants and plant products was started by our ancestors for the purpose of disease treatment. Similarly, many plants were traditionally used to treat liver toxicity and other liver diseases. Some of the plants that have liver protective effects are mentioned below-

Trailing Eclipta Leaf and Root (*Eclipta alba*) - Demethylwedelolactone and wedelolactone are the two coumestans isolated from streaming eclipta as major active compounds. In the cultured rat hepatocytes using liver enzyme-induced cytotoxicity, these two components had shown anti-hepatotoxic properties. These ingredients also had shown an effect on the regeneration of liver cells [11].

Long pepper Fruit (*Piper longum*) - Piperine is an active constituent that has shown hepatoprotective activity against the toxicity induced by carbon tetrachloride and tertiary butyl hydroperoxide. It reduces the decrease in glutathione (GSH) both *in-vitro* and *in-vivo* by lipid peroxidation [11].

Andographis Aerial Parts (*Andographis paniculata*) – Traditionally, it is used as hepatoprotective against hepatotoxicity and for various liver disorders. The increase in glutathione is due to the andographis and diterpenes that can reduce oxidative tissue damage [11].

Ginger Rhizome (*Zingiber officinale*) – Digestion is traditionally promoted by ginger. It is found to have a reviving effect on gastric secretions. In conjugation with other herbs, it shows a metabolic circulatory reviving effect.

Embelia Fruit (*Embelia ribes*) – Traditionally, this fruit is used to rejuvenate the liver as well as other liver ailments.

Arjuna Myrobalan Bark (*Terminalia arjuna*) – Traditionally, it was used for the treatment of liver cirrhosis as a general tonic and diuretic.

Hellebore Root (*Helleborus viridis*) – Traditionally, it was used in combatting hepatitis, fever, poisoning, liver cleansing, and as a liver tonic. It has no side effects. Recent studies also have shown that its roots can be used against alcohol-induced hepatotoxicity.

Neem (*Azadirachta indica*) – Neem is a member of the Meliaceae family of plants. It is useful against constipation, intestinal worm, leprosy, skin infections, anorexia, blood morbidity and biliary affliction. The plant has bitter active constituents in different parts [11]. The hepatoprotective activity of alcoholic, aqueous, petroleum ether, and ethyl extract of the leaves has been reported [11]. In the hepatic damage due to carbon tetrachloride, the juice of young stem bark shows hepatoprotective as well as antioxidant properties [12]. In rats, hepatic damage caused by paracetamol can be treated with the leaves, showing a hepatoprotective effect [11].

Tulsi (*Ocimum sanctum*) – *Ocimum sanctum* belongs to the Lamiaceae family and has a wide range of therapeutic activities. It is a popular remedy for stomach disorders, malaria, inflammation and heart disease. The hepatoprotective potential of this plant is reported against carbon tetrachloride, paracetamol, and lead-induced liver damage [13, 14].

Turmeric (*Curcuma longa*) – It is a member of the Zingiberaceae family and it is widely known as turmeric or haldi. The juice of the rhizome is useful for the treatment of various diseases. These include asthma, anthelmintic, urinary infections, gonorrhoea, *etc.* The essential oil present in *Curcuma longa* is used as stomachic, carminative and tonic [15, 16]. Traditionally, *Curcuma longa* is also used in the treatment of several liver disorders including liver cirrhosis [17]. It shows hepatoprotective activity against hepatotoxicity induced by carbon tetrachloride and thioacetamide [11, 18]. Its hepatoprotective property is contributed by its anti-inflammatory and antioxidant properties [19, 20]. Salt of curcumin which is known as sodium curcuminate can accelerate the excretion of bilirubin, bile salts and cholesterol through the bile, thus treating cholelithiasis. It has exhibited no toxic effect up to 2.5 g/kg body weight [21]. In humans, high doses of *Curcuma longa* may cause gastric irritation.

Fenugreek (*Trigonella foenum-graecum*) – It is commonly known as fenugreek or methi and it belongs to the Fabaceae family. Fenugreek leaves can be used in the treatment of liver diseases and can be included as a dietary supplement due to their antioxidant, cytoprotective and hepatoprotective activity [22]. It has been reported that liver toxicity induced by deltamethrin can be protected by the oxidative property of *Trigonella* [22]. Increased GSH, Lipid peroxidation (LPO) content and decreased activity of antioxidants *i.e* GST, Superoxide dismutases (SOD) and catalase were detected in rat liver due to oxidative stress induced by deltamethrin. *Trigonella* also has antilipidemic and antioxidative properties. It shows activity against toxicity induced by pesticides. For carbon tetrachloride - induced toxicity, the methanol extract of *Trigonella* can be used [23]. Liver cirrhosis induced by thioacetamide can also be treated with the dried seed extract of *Trigonella* [24].

Indian Gall Fruit (*Terminalia chebula*) – *Terminalia chebula* is commonly known as Myrobalan, belonging to the Combretaceae family. Traditionally, it is used for dysentery, chronic diarrhoea, and enlarged liver and spleen. It can also be used to prevent and treat liver damage because it scavenges free radicals. It also helps in the treatment of hepatitis, jaundice and fatty liver. It has hypercholesterolemic activity and hypercholesterolemia induced by cholesterol.

Henna (*Lawsonia inermis*) – *Lawsonia inermis*, which is commonly known as henna belongs to the Lythraceae family. This plant is used in medicine as a coagulant for open wounds, among other uses. Fresh leaves of henna are used as an antiseptic for bacterial and fungal skin infections. It can also improve the health of the hair. Furthermore, it is traditionally used in the treatment of liver diseases such as liver enlargement and jaundice through the usage of a tree bark.

Turpeth (*Operculina turpethum*) – It belongs to the family of Convolvulaceae. In Ayurveda, the treatment of jaundice is initiated with the remedy of turpeth. It is usually given in a powdered form of about 1 to 2 teaspoons in warm water, twice a day.

Dandelion (*Taraxacum officinale*) – It revives the gall bladder and the liver for appropriate exertion of fats in the body. It is beneficial in detoxifying the liver. The juice is beneficial in the treatment of various liver problems. Dandelion tea is also beneficial for hepatitis patients.

Capillary Wormwood *(Artemisia scoparia)* -*Artemisia scoparia* belongs to the daisy family and has a hepatoprotective effect. The hydroalcoholic extract of Artemisia scoparia provides hepatoprotective activity against liver damage that is caused by acetaminophen and carbon tetrachloride. The administered dose decreased hepatotoxin that was induced by biochemical parameters *i.e.* increased serum levels alanine transferase (ALT) and aspartate transaminase (AST) and improved phenobarbital-induced sleep duration, indicating hepatoprotective effect. Paracetamol and carbon tetrachloride decrease the activity of enzymes that metabolise the drug, slowing down drug metabolism, and resulting in improved concentration of drugs such as barbiturates, which prolong the pharmacological effects such as sleep duration. Hepatoprotective activity is suggested by the reversal of sleep time induced by barbiturates. The hepatoprotective activity is supported by antioxidant and anti-inflammatory activity [25, 26].

Egyptian Balsam *(Balanites aegyptiaca)* - It belongs to the Zygophyllaceae family. It shows activity against hepatoxicity induced by carbon tetrachloride and paracetamol [27, 28]. It decreases the biochemical *i.e* serum ALT, AST, alkaline phosphatase (ALP) and bilirubin induced by hepatotoxin. Moreover, it reverses the improved ratio of sleep duration induced by pentobarbital. It also has anti-inflammatory, and antioxidant properties, thereby improving the hepatoprotective effect [29].

Marshworts *(Apium graveolens)* - It belongs to the Apiaceae family. Hepatoxicity induced by paracetamol and carbon tetrachloride can be treated by the methanolic extract of *Apium graveolens*. The dose attenuated the biochemicals *i.e* serum activated partial thromboplastin time (APT), AST, ALT albumin and total proteins induced by the hepatotoxin and histopathological change in liver tissue. No adverse symptoms for acute toxicity are reported. Lethal dose was found to be 7.5 gm/kg weight in 50% of rats, showing a wide safety margin [30].

Brahmi *(Bacopa monnieri)*- It belongs to the Plantaginaceae family. The ethanolic extract of *Bacopa monnieri* gives hepatoprotective action against liver damage induced by morphine and nitrobenzene [31, 32]. The dose attenuated the biochemicals *i.e* serum APT, AST and histopathological changes. It also has antioxidant and anti-inflammatory activity which thereby improves hepatoprotective activity. The single LD_{50} dose was established to be 2400 mg/kg body weight of rats. In chronic toxicity, upto 500 mg/kg body weight for 3 months was well tolerated [33].

Beetroot *(Beta vulgaris)*-*Beta vulgaris* belongs to the family of Amaranthaceae. The ethanolic extract of *Beta vulgaris* roots showed dose-dependent hepatoprotective efficacy against carbon tetrachloride-induced liver injury [34]. The anti-inflammatory and antioxidant properties of the compound may be responsible for this hepatoprotective activity [35]. This plant is tolerated even at high doses.

Tea Plant *(Camellia sinensis)*-*Camellia sinensis* belongs to the Theaceae family. An aqueous extract of *Camellia sinensis* showed hepatoprotective properties against carbon tetrachloride induced liver damage in rats. The extract decreased the dose of biochemical substances, *i.e.*, AST, ALP, ALT, albumin, and total protein, as well as the histopathological changes of the liver [36]. It possesses certain anti-inflammatory, antioxidant, and immunomodulatory activities which attribute to hepatoprotective activity [37]. High doses of this tea show stimulation of the CNS due to the presence of caffeine.

Arabian Balsam Tree *(Commiphora opobalsamum)* - It belongs to the family of Burseraceae. The ethanolic extract of *Commiphora opobalasum* showed hepatoprotective behaviour against carbon tetrachloride-induced liver damage. It provides attenuated biochemicals such as serum ALT, AST, AST and prolonged barbiturate sleeping time. The hepatoprotective behaviour is contributed by prominent anti-inflammatory and antioxidant activity.

Red Spiderling *(Boerhaavia diffusa)*-*Boerhaavia diffusa* belongs to the family Nyctaginaceae. Its ethanolic aqueous extract lessened ethanol and acetaminophen-induced biochemicals *i.e* rise of serum ALT, AST, bilirubin, APT and histopathological changes in the liver [38, 39]. This shows the hepatoprotective behaviour of the extract. The oral LD_{50} dose in rats and mice was 2000mg/kg body weight [40].

Asian Pigeonwings *(Clitoria ternatea)*–*Clitoria ternatea* belongs to the family of Fabaceae. The seeds, leaves, and flowers are traditionally used against liver diseases [41]. Liver damage induced by hepatotoxins such as paracetamol and carbon tetrachloride could be attenuated by the methanolic extract of *Clitoria ternatea*. Hepatoprotective activities are indicated by decreased biochemicals such as serum AST, ALT, and bilirubin levels as well as histological changes in the liver. The antioxidant and anti-inflammatory activity contributes to hepatoprotective effects. The LD_{50} dose was found to be 3000 mg/kg body weight [41].

Ficus Tree *(Ficus Carica)*-*Ficus Carica* is part of the family of Moraceae. Its hepatoprotective activity is seen against rifampicin and carbon tetrachloride-induced toxicity [42, 43]. Its hepatoprotective activity is contributed by its antioxidant and anti-inflammatory activity. Generally, the well-ripened fruit is considered safe but unripe fruit may have toxic effects and can cause contact dermatitis [44].

Phalsa Cherry *(Grewia tenax)* - It belongs to the family of Malvaceae. Its roots, leaves and fruits are used in the treatment of jaundice, digestive problem and inflammatory conditions [45]. Carbon tetrachloride-induced hepatotoxicity causes a marked increase in biochemical *i.e.* serum ALT, total bilirubin (TB), AST, APT, and gamma-glutamyl transferase and also contributes to the histopathology alteration in rats which can be reversed by giving ethanolic extract of *Greawiatenax*. Its hepatoprotective activity can also be suggested by the reversing in prolongation of narcolepsy induced by pentobarbital. Its chronic administration reduces low-density lipoprotein (LDL); cholesterol and triglycerides levels [46]. It shows adverse effects such as mild diarrhoea in doses of more than 2 g/kg body weight of mice. The anti-inflammatory and antioxidant activity contributes to hepatoprotective activity.

Mediterranean Heath *(Erica multiflora)* - It belongs to the family of Ericaceae. It is used to treat intestinal and liver disorders. Medicinal constituents of the plant are its seeds and leaves, which have hepatoprotective, antioxidant and anti-inflammatory activity [47]. An ethanolic extract of the seeds and leaves showed activity against liver damage caused by ethanol and carbon tetrachloride [47, 48]. A cytoprotective effect is also observed on liver cancer cells. The plant is edible and there is no toxicity reported so far.

Fruiting Branch *(Grewia mollis)-* It is from the family of Malvaceae. It is used in the treatment of abdominal issues, liver disorders and inflammatory conditions and arthritis [49]. The methanolic extract of *Grewia mollis* was found to have hepatoprotective activity against carbon tetrachloride-induced liver injury [50]. Its anti-inflammatory and antioxidant properties may contribute to its hepatoprotective properties [50].

Garden Cress *(Lepidium sativum)* - It belongs to the family of Brassicaceae. *Lepidium sativum* and is used for liver problems such as jaundice, spleen diseases, arthritis, gastrointestinal disorder, and inflammatory conditions. The methanolic extract has caused hepatoprotective activity against liver injury in rats induced by carbon tetrachloride. The dose lessened the rise in biochemicals *i.e.* ALT, APT, AST and bilirubin, indicating hepatoprotective activity [51]. Its anti-inflammatory and antioxidant properties could contribute to the hepatoprotective effect. 2% w/w in the diet of rats had shown no toxicity but 10% w/w had shown mild toxicity [52].

Plants contain various types of secondary metabolites. These phytoconstituents confer different pharmacological activities. Table **1** illustrates detailed information on the phytoactive components and the summary of the mode of action of the hepatoprotective activity of the medicinal plant.

Table 1. Details of Bioactive components and mode of action of hepatoprotective activity of medicinal plants.

Biological sources	Vernacular name	Family	Part used	Extract used	Chief bioactive components	The pharmacological screening model used	Summary of mode of action of biochemical parameters and histopathological analysis studied	Refs
Curcuma longa	Turmeric	Zingiberaceae	Rhizome	Ethanolic	Curcumin, bisdemethoxycurcumin, turmerone, demethoxycurcumin, curcuphenol, cyclocurcumin	Liver injury induced by ethanol	Provides a molecular platform for its application in hepatic disorders.	[53]
Silybum marianum	Milk thistle	Asteraceae	Seed	Ethanol	Isosilychristin, Isosilibinin, silybin A, isosilybin A, silydianin, silybin B, isosilybin B and silychristin.	Liver injury caused by carbon tetrachloride, radiation, acetaminophen, alcohol, and phenyl hydrazine	It works as an antioxidant by lowering lipid peroxidation and free radical generation, as well as having antifibrotic properties and perhaps acting as a toxin blocker by preventing toxins from attaching to hepatocyte cell membrane receptors.	[54]
Phyllanthus amarus	Bhumi amlaki	Phyllanthaceae	Seed	Ethanolic	Phyllanthin, hypophyllanthin, nirphyllin, phyllanthin, phyltetralinphyllangin, and phyllnirurin	Rat liver cell injury induced by ethanol	Phyllanthin proved its protective function by combatting the ethanol-induced impact.	[55]
Glycyrrhiza glabra	Licorice	Fabaceae	Root	Ethanol	Glycyrrhizin, licoisoflavanone, liocflavanol, glabroisoflavanone, licoricone, liquiritigenin,rhamnolliuiritin, gralbraninand gancaonin	Hepatotoxicity induced by acetaminophen in mature Sprague Dawley rats model	In order to preserve liver function and prevent hepatocellular cancer, it lessens the amount and magnitude of GT-positive foci.	[56]

(Table 1) cont.....

Biological sources	Vernacular name	Family	Part used	Extract used	Chief bioactive components	The pharmacological screening model used	Summary of mode of action of biochemical parameters and histopathological analysis studied	Refs
Gentiana olivieri	Gulechafis	Gentianaceae	Flowering herbs	Ethyl acetate	Isoorientin, Iridoids, oliverine, Isoorientin, gentianine, olvieramine, gentioflavin, olivieridine, and gentianidine	CCl_4 induced hepatic damage in rat	Non-protein cysteine reservoir in the liver is involved in many cellular processes including the detoxification of the liver.	[57]
Rubia cordifolia	Mungistarox	Rubiaceae	Root and stem	Ethanolic	Rubiadin, pseudopurpurin, munjistin, 1,3-dimethoxy 2-carboxy anthraquinone and 1,4-dihydroxy 2-methyl anthraquinone	Hepatic damage induced by CCl_4	Rubiadin also substantially decreased glutathione levels and hepatic malondialdehyde production in the liver of CCl_4 induced toxicity in a dose-dependent manner.	[58]
Brazilian propolis	Bitter root	---	Pollen	Methanolic	3-hydroxy-2,2-dimethyl-8-prenychromane-6-propenoic acid, Galangin, quercetin, kaemferol, chrysin, pinocembrine and saccharin	On TNF-α/D-GaIN induced cell death in primary cultured mouse hepatocytes	The phenolic components in tropical *Brazilian propolis* alcoholic extract, particularly flavonoids, are primarily responsible for its hepatoprotective properties.	[59]
Clitoria ternatea	Cordofanpea	Fabaceae	Flower	Methanolic	Kaempferol, kaempferol 3-2 Grhamnosylrutinoside, kaempferol 3-neohesperidoside	Acetaminophen induced liver damage	Total phenolics and flavonoids were estimated to be 105.40 ± 2.47 mg/g gallic acid equivalent and 72.21 ± 0.05 mg/g catechin equivalent.	[60]
Cochlospermum vitifolium	Aconitum vitifolium	Bixaceae	Stem bark	Ethyl acetate	Naringenin, dihydrocochloxanthin, antiarol, vitixanthin, 7,4'-dimethoxytaxifolin and dihydrovitixanthin	Liver injury induced by 35 mg/kg of phenobarbital *i.pin* rat	To evaluate its hepatoprotective effect, it was given to rats with obstructed bile ducts.	[61]
Schouwia thebaica	Marsh	Brassicaceae	Aerial part	Alcoholic	Chrysoeriol-7-O-xylosoide-(1,2)-arabinofuranoside	CCl_4 treated rats	After limiting the secretion of hepatic triglycerides into plasma, these benefits are attributed to the buildup of triglycerides in hepatocytes.	[62]
Rubus alceifolius	Raspberries, blackberries, addewberries	Rosaceae	Flower	Ethanolic	1-2-3-hydroxyeuscaphic acid, gallic acid and ellagic acid	Liver injury induced by CCl_4 in mice	When comparing the fraction, the low-dose ethyl acetate fraction proved the most active. AST and ALT were found to be lowered; hepatic MDA and NO were prevented, and SOD was increased.	[63]
Clausena lansium	Wampee	Rutaceae	Stem bark	Methanolic	Mauritianin, dihydrofuranocoumarin glycosides, adenosine, Imperatorin and chalepin	CCl_4 induced hepatotoxicity	When serum liver proteins are increased by 7.0-8.8% and AST, ALT, and ALP activity by 27.7-107.9%, serum liver protein levels are restored.	[64]
Solanum fastigiatum	Jambolao	Solanaceae	Whole plant	Aqueous	Quercetin and rutin	Paracetamol induced liver necrosis in mice	An enzyme assay showed hepatoprotective action, reversing the changes in thiobarbituric acid reactive compounds.	[65]
Padina boergesenii	Brown algae	Dictyotaceae	Seaweed	Diethyl ether	Fucoxanthin, phenolic compounds, sterol, monoterpenes, and carotenoid	Oxidative damage induced by CCl_4 in Wistar rats	Researchers are currently working to isolate and identify bioactive components from *P. boergesenii* in order to determine the possible mechanism of liver protection.	[66]
Phyllanthus acidus	Malay gooseberry	Phyllanthaceae	Leaf fruit	Ethane	Quercetin, kaempferol, gallic acid, hypogallicacid, adenosine, α-cadinol, β-cadinene, t-muurolol and α-muurolene	Hepatic damage was caused by thioacetamide and acetaminophen in Wistar rats	The presence of TAA in the above serum parameters indicates that it has hepatoprotective properties.	[67]
Castanea crenata	Jepanese chestnut	Fagaceae	Chestnut	Methanolic	Scoparone, scopoletin, hydrolysable tannins, ellagic, gallic acids Kurigalin and agallotannin	In C57BL/6 mice, chronic ethanol exposure caused oxidative damage	Enhancement of the liver's antioxidant defence mechanism via inhibiting lipid buildup and peroxidation.	[68]
Hydrocotyle sibthorpioides	Bakongrimba	Araliaceae	Entire plant	Ethanolic	Asiaticoside, quercetin, daucosterol, isorhamnetin, quercetin 3-O-β-D-(6-caffeoylgalactoside), genistein, demecolcine, stigmasterol, quercetin 3-galactoside and daidzein	Five HBV promoters in HepG2.2.15 cells	By suppressing the actions of the core, s1,s2, and X gene promoters, viral DNA transcription and replication were diminished.	[69]
Fumaria indica	Indian fumitory	Papaveraceae	Arial plant	Methanolic	Monomethyl fumarate, protopine, bicuculine, narceimine, fumariline, oxyhydrastinine, fumarilicine and oxysanguinarine	Rifampicin, paracetamol, and CCl_4 induce liver toxicity	There's a possibility that monomethyl fumarate antihepatotoxic efficacy against rifampicin is attributed to suppression of the active metabolite, 25 desacetylrifampin.	[70]
Antrodia camphorata	Camphoratakanehirai	Polyporaceae	Fruiting bodies	Fermented filtration of Niuchangchih	Antrocin, antrocamphin A, antrocinnamomins A, ergostatrien-3β-ol, Lignans, ergosterol peroxide, Lanostane, Succinic and hexadecanoic acid	Liver damage induced by cytokine and CCl_4 in mice	In this way, free radical damage to cells can be prevented, and the antioxidant enzymes can be enhanced.	[71]

(Table 1) cont.....

Biological sources	Vernacular name	Family	Part used	Extract used	Chief bioactive components	The pharmacological screening model used	Summary of mode of action of biochemical parameters and histopathological analysis studied	Refs
Rosemarinus officinalis	Rosemary	Lamiaceae	Leaf	Ethanolic	Carnosic acid, caffeic acid, rosmarinic acid, chlorogenic acid, monomeric acid, carnosol, oleanolic acid, carnosic acid, alpha-pinene, camphor, eucalyptol, rosmadial, rosmanol and ursolic acid	Azathioprine induced toxicity in rats	Extracts to inhibit the proliferation of human liver carcinoma cells.	[72]
Physalis peruviana	Cape goose berry	Solanaceae	Leaf and root	Ethane, water, hexane	28-hydroxywithanolide, withanolides, phygrine and kaempferol	In rats, CCl_4 caused acute liver damage	The antioxidant property is claimed to be one of the mechanisms of hepatoprotective effects	[73]
Panax ginseng	Ginseng	Araliaceae	Aerial parts	Ethanolic	Ginsenosides, panaxosides, polyacetylenic alcohols and oleanane	In rats, CCl_4 caused liver damage	Honey's and Korrean ginseng extract's protective qualities could be linked to their antioxidant capacity.	[74]
Eclipta prostrata	Bringaraj	Asteraceae	Whole plant	80% methanol	Echinocystic acid, wedelolactone, β-amyrin, heptacosanol, hentriacontano, demethylw-edelolactone and demethylwedelolactone-7-glucoside	HSCs (hepatic stellate cells) have long been thought to contribute in the development of liver fibrosis.	Utilizing the HSC-T6 cell line from rat liver, as an in vitro test method, to determine the activity of natural products.	[75]
Rhus verniciflua	Chinese lacquer tree	Anacardiaceae	Stem bark	Ethanolic	Glycoprotein (36 kDa), gallic acid, methyl gallate, butin, sulfuretin, catechol and kaempferol	CCl_4 induced liver injury in mice	It is hypothesised that the RVS glycoprotein safeguards the liver from injury by eliminating radicals.	[76]
Crateva nurvala	Sungrass	Capparaceae	Root	Ethanolic	Lupeol, lupeol linoleate, pentacyclic triterpenoid, kaemferol, dodecanoic anhydride, quercitin, friedelin, betulinic acid, rutin and cadabicine	Cadmium induced hepatotoxicity in rats	Free radical removal and improvement of the liver antioxidant state are two ways to combat free radicals.	[77]
Achillea millefolium	Gandrain yarrow	Asteraceae	Whole herb	20% methanolic	Luteolin-7-O-b-D-glucoronide, longifolene, chamazulene, isoborneol, camphor and Dicaffeoylquinic acids (DCCAs)	In the isolate perfused rat liver	DCCAs and luteolin-7--b-D-glucoronide combination to increase bile circulation greater efficiently than cynarin alone.	[78]
Momordica dioica Roxb.	Spiny gourd	Cucurbitaceae	Leaves	Aqueous and ethanolic	6-methyl tritriacont-5-on-28 ol, and 8-methyl hentriacont-3-ene, and momordicaursenol	CCl_4 induced hepatotoxicity in rats	Lowers the levels of SALP, SGOT, SGPT, and total bilirubin in serum	[79]
Asparagus racemosus	Shatavari	Liliaceae	Whole plant	Aqueous fraction and crude extract	Asparagamine A, Shatvarin, rutin, Immunoside, dihydrophenantherene, quercitin andhyperoside	γ-radiation induced liver injury	Lowers protein oxidation and lipid peroxidation	[80]
Luffa echinata	Bindal	Cucurbitaceae	Fruits	Acetone, petroleum ether, and methanolic extract	Hentriacontane, sapogenin, coumaric acid, cucurbitacin E, eletarin-2-glucoside and echinatin	CCl_4 induced liver injury	Lowers the levels of total albumin, total protein, SGPT, and SGOT	[81]
Aloe barbadensis	Aloe vera	Asphodelaceae	Dried aerial parts	Methanolic, petroleum ether, and chloroform extract	Aloe-emodin, feralolide, chromones, Anthraquinones, tannin and phlobatannins	CCl_4 induced liver injury	Lowers the level of bilirubin, serum transaminase, microsomal aniline hydroxylase, lipid peroxidation, and triglycerides in serum.	[82]
Cassia tora	Sickle senna	Fabaceae	Leaves	Ethyl acetate fraction	Geraniol, nerol, and terpinen-4-ol	CCl_4 induced liver injury	Reduced glutathione enzyme activities.	[83]
Acacia catechu	Khair	Leguminosae	Powdered pale catechu	Ethyl acetate fraction	Kaempferol, 4-hydroxybenzoic acid	CCl_4 induced liver injury	Lowers the levels of total bilirubin, SGOT, and SGPT in serum.	[84]
Tylophora indica	Antamool	Asclepiadaceae	Powder leaf	Aqueous fraction	Tylophorine, kaempferol, quercetin, hydroxyisotylocrebrine and tetratriacontanol	Ethanol induced liver injury	Reduced the levels of total bilirubin. ALP, AST, and ALT	[85]
Alocasia indica	Giant taro	Araceae	Leaves	Hydroalcoholic extract	Lutein, glycosides, β-carotene, flavonoids, succinic acid, cynogeneticalocasin, amino acids, and β-lectins	Paracetamol induced hepatotoxicity	Reduced the levels of AST, ALP, ALT, and total bilirubin in serum.	[86]
Acacia confusa	Pilampwoia	Fabaceae	Bark	Hydroalcoholic extract	N-methyltryptamine, oxalyldiaminopropionic acid	CCl_4 induced liver injury	Lowers the levels of MDA, SOD, ALT, AST, CAT and GPx in erythrocytes	[87]
Carum copticum	Thymol seeds	Apiaceae	Seed	Water	Thymol, o-cymene, carvacrol, γ-terpinene and nerolidol	CCl_4 and paracetamol induced liver injury	Lowers the levels of ALP, ALT, AST, and serum glutamic-pyruvic transaminase in serum.	[88]
Hypericum japonicum	St. Jhon's-wort	Hypericaceae	Whole plant	Aqueous, chloroform, and petroleum ether	JaponicinA,B,C, and D, Quercetin, Kaempferol, rutin, Sarothranol, Sarothralin and Isojacareubin	α-naphthyl-isothiocyanate and CCl_4 induced liver injury	Lowers the levels of total bilirubin, ALP, ALT, and AST in serum.	[89]
Euphorbia fusiformis	Asthma plant	Euphorbiaceae	Tubers	Ethanolic extract	Afzelin, euphorbin-C, heptacosane, chtolphenolic acid	Rifampicin induced liver injury	Lowers the levels of total bilirubin, GGTP, SGOT, SGPT in serum.	[90]
Bupleurum kaoi	Chinese thoroughwax	Apiaceae	Dried roots	Ethanolic extract	Borneol, neral, oleananelignins, phenyl propanol derivatives and myrtenol	CCl_4 induced liver injury	Lowers the levels of ALP, SGPT, SGOT, and histopathological studies.	[91]
Laggera pterodonta	Curly blumea	Asteraceae	Whole herb	Aqueous and ethyl alcohol extract	Ilicic acid, patuletin, pterodondiol, chrysosplenetin, chrysosplenetin B and tamarixetin	D- galactosamine and CCl_4 induced liver injury	Lowers the levels of total bilirubin, ALP, ALT, and AST in serum.	[92]

IMPROVED HEPATOPROTECTIVE EFFICACY OF HERBAL DRUGS USING NANO-BASED DRUG DELIVERY SYSTEMS

Many herbal extracts/drugs have a broad range of medicinal properties. However, due to their poor absorption and bioavailability after oral administration, the prospective application of these herbal medications is limited. The bioavailability can be improved by novel drug delivery systems which can enhance the rate and extent of solubilisation of the drug in aqueous intestinal fluids as well as the capacity to cross the lipid-rich biological membranes. For this purpose, the formulation of novel drug delivery systems and carriers with herbal drugs/extracts should preferably fulfill some essential criteria. These include proper drug delivery at a rate oriented by the body's needs over the course of treatment and passing the active ingredient of the herbal drug to the target site [93]. A variety of techniques have been used to improve the solubility, shelf life, bioavailability and gastrointestinal permeability of the drugs [94]. Nanocarriers have received much attention in the development of innovative pharmaceutical carriers and delivery methods. Encapsulation of herbal extracts and metabolites into biodegradable and biocompatible nanocarriers is one strategy to overcome this difficulty [95]. On the other hand, bioavailability can be improved by increasing the frequency and volume of solubility of the drug in aqueous intestinal fluids along with transportability in lipid-based biological membranes. The encapsulation of herbal extracts/drugs in novel carrier systems solves the limitations associated with the physiochemical and pharmacokinetic activity of phytoconstituents. This breakthrough indicates a bright future for nanomedicine as a potential option to overcome and treat a wide range of chronic diseases [96]. Moreover, the use of alternative nanocarriers such as organic, inorganic, or hybrid carriers of different sizes and shapes, as well as surface modification approaches such as the addition of charges and functional groups, PEGylation, or ligands, are expected to be an important factor in tuning their physiochemical properties. The main goal of using nanocarriers in drug delivery is to successfully treat a disease with as minimal adverse effects and outcomes as possible [97]. Table **2** shows the list of nano-based drug carriers of natural products with hepatoprotective activity.

Table 2. Novel drug delivery of natural products having hepatoprotective activity.

Delivery system/carrier	Phytoconstituent/extract	Effects	Ref
Self-nanoemulsifying drug delivery systems (SNEDDSs)	*Beta vulgaris* Leaves extract (beetroot) have phenolic acids, carotenoids, and flavonoids.	Shown significantly improved hepatoprotective activity in thioacetamide-induced hepatotoxicity in rats and also improved liver function parameters and inflammatory markers as compared to the plain extract.	[98]

(Table 2) cont.....

Delivery system/carrier	Phytoconstituent/extract	Effects	Ref
Nanoparticles	*Cuscuta chinensis* seeds extract have flavonoids and lignans.	Showed improved hepatoprotective and antioxidant activity in acetaminophen-induced hepatotoxicity in rats and required less dose in NPs loaded with cuscuta extract as compared to plain extract.	[99]
Nanoemulsion	Leaves and berries extract of *Phyllanthus amarus*	Nanoencapsulated ethanolic extract of *Phyllanthus amarus* induces significant hepatoprotective effect in carbon tetrachloride induced hepatotoxicity in rats.	[100]
Liposomes	*Orthosiphon stamineus* leaves ethanolic extract	Provide enhanced solubility, absorption, antioxidant hepatoprotective effect in thioacetamide-induced liver cirrhosis in rats.	[101]
Herbosomes	*Andrographis paniculate* extract andrographolides	Andrographolide herbosome resolves rapid clearance and low elimination half-life problem and provides significant protection to the liver of rats, restoring hepatic enzyme activity in carbon tetrachloride-treated rats.	[102]
Lipid-polymer hybrid nanoparticles	β-Sitosterol (BSS) phytosterol extract from dried and powered arial parts of *Centaurea pumilio*	This formulation is significantly able to restore normal liver structure and functioning as well as reduce the cleaved caspase-3 expression which is responsible for hepatotoxic effect and found to be hopeful hepatoprotective drug delivery system.	[103]
Silver nanoparticles	*Azima tetracantha* extract	Prepared nanoparticles significantly restore normal liver structure and provide hepatoprotective effects.	[104]
Silver nanoparticles	Shade-dried *Rhizophora apiculata* leaf extract	Provide protective effect on the liver in carbon tetrachloride-treated rats.	[105]
Nanoemulsion	Silymarin	Poorly water-soluble silymarin-loaded nanoemulsion provides excellent hepatic protection.	[106]
Liposomes	Silibinin	Provide hepatoprotection and antiulcer activity.	[107]

MEDICINAL PLANTS SHOWING HEPATOTOXICITY ACTIVITY

Atractylis gummifera

There are more than 26 species of thistle in the Mediterranean province, including *Atractylis gummifera*. Although carboxyatractyloside and atractyloside, which are abundant in the root of the plant, are known to be toxic, *A. gummifera* continues to be eaten [108, 109]. By taking into account a mitochondrial enzyme called adenine nucleotide translocator, these two diterpenoid glucosides, namely carboxyatractyloside and atractyloside, can interfere with mitochondrial energy metabolism [109]. In addition, toxicity associated with dermal exposure has been noted [110]. In vitro studies have revealed that certain drugs such as dithiothreitol or verapamil, may protect against atractyloside poisoning by impeding adenosine diphosphate-adenosine tri-phosphate synthesis through P450 cytochrome suppression, only when it is administered prior to atractyloside [111].

Callilepsis laureola

The Zulu tribe has historically used a native plant to the vicinity of Natal in South Africa called *Callilepsis laureola* as a traditional remedy [112]. However, numerous cases of acute renal and hepatic dysfunction have been documented with a death rate of more than 90% within 5 days [113]. Interestingly, *C. laureola* causes cytotoxicity in Hep G2 (human hepatoma cells) by decreasing cellular glutathione content. It has been shown that this cytotoxicity can be reduced by loading the cells with N-acetylcysteine to avoid glutathione depletion [114].

Larrea tridentate

Larrea tridentate (Chaparral) is a species native to Mexico and the southwestern United States [108]. It has been used to alleviate a variety of ailments, including bronchitis, cancer, pain and skin diseases as well as an alternative therapy for acquired immune deficiency syndrome [115]. The consumption of chaparral herb has been associated with a number of reports on liver damage, particularly cholestatic hepatitis and acute and subacute hepatocellular injury [116]. In 1997, Sheikh *et al.* reviewed 13 cases of liver injury caused by chaparral. Numerous subjects had developed jaundice and significant serum elevation at ALT after 3 to 52 weeks of use; this condition often disappeared 1 to 17 weeks after discontinuation of the drug. In addition, liver cirrhosis later developed in 4 subjects while liver transplantation was required in 2 subjects due to acute liver failure [117]. Histopathological observations, particularly in zone 3, included extensive liver necrosis and changes in bile and cholestasis [118, 119].

Teucrium chamaedrys

Teucrium chamaedrys (Germander) is a species belonging to the native of Middle East and Europe and it is used to treat obesity, gout, dyspepsia, diabetes and hypertension [120]. There are several cases of liver destruction (especially in France), some of which have manifested as acute liver failure, and acute and chronic hepatitis [121, 122]. Most episodes of hepatotoxicity occurred after two months of taking the drug at the manufacturer's recommended dosage (600-1600 mg/day) [123]. In addition to general symptoms such as nausea, jaundice, anorexia and gastric discomfort, there was a significant increase in ALT. Jaundice usually resolved within 8 weeks after discontinuation. However, isolated reports of cirrhosis and relapse after accidental exposure have been documented [122].

Chelidonium majus

Chelidonium majus (Greater celandine) is a European plant that contains at least 20 different alkaloids, including chelerythrine, chelidonine, berberine, chelerythrine and coptisine. Its preparations are used to relieve irritable bowel syndrome and bilious complaints [120]. The largest case series, which included 10 female patients had mild ALP and ALT elevations that often began 3 months after ingestion [124]. Five subjects had visible cholestasis but did not develop liver failure. The majority of liver biopsies revealed eosinophilic nodules and portal dysfunction. In most subjects, discontinuation of the elevated celandine medication resulted in the recovery of liver biochemical analysis within 2 to 6 months.

FUTURE PROSPECT

Since ancient times, plants have been used for medicinal purposes to treat various ailments. Today, the demand for natural phytochemicals from plants is on the rise. To meet this demand, plants must be cloned in large quantities using tissue culture techniques. While conventional methods might take up a long time, in vitro methods can be used to rapidly generate large numbers of medicinal plants and active metabolites. Therefore, biotechnological expertise offers good opportunities for the development of in vitro production of medicinal plants.

Allopathic drugs are available to cure diseases but they are usually expensive and have limited efficacy. In addition, they show adverse effects in many cases. However, it is certain that herbal medicines have no adverse effects. They are inexpensive and do not show adverse effects even when they are consumed for a long period. Since modern medicine does not provide effective therapy for chronic diseases and multidrug-resistant pathogens and parasites, the use of traditional medicines has greatly increased in industrialised countries. Various medicinal plants have hepatoprotective effects and help to protect and heal liver damage. Nowadays, allopathic medicines are being replaced by traditional herbal medicines to cure liver problems. In many developed and developing countries, the use of allopathic medicines to cure liver diseases has been reduced to a certain level. However, herbal formulations can be improved by using a novel drug delivery technology and currently, there are many studies being conducted in the pharmaceutical industry to produce new herbal formulations.

CONCLUSION

Modern society has inherited the knowledge of medicinal treatment of liver injuries from various cultures. A majority of herbal medicines including turmeric, licorice, green tea and milk thistle are well-known plants for the treatment of liver disease. Studies have shown that various parts of medicinal plants can be used for liver diseases. These plants offer alternatives to the limited therapeutic options offered by allopathic drugs for hepatotoxins. One of the findings is that most medicinal plants have anti-inflammatory and antioxidant properties, which contribute to the hepatoprotective nature of the plant. Herbal treatments are safe and effective.

REFERENCES

[1]   Andreoli, T.; Carpenter, C.J.; Griggs, R.; Benjamin, I. Diseases of the Liver and Biliary System. Andreoli, TE; Carpenter, CCJ & La Fayette Cecil, R Cecil's Essentials of Medicine. Saunders: Philadelphia, **2007**.

[2]   Rashmi, R.; Bojan Magesh, S.; Mohanram Ramkumar, K.; Suryanarayanan, S.; Venkata SubbaRao, M.; SubbaRao, MV. Antioxidant potential of naringenin helps to protect liver tissue from streptozotocin-induced damage. *Rep. Biochem. Mol. Biol.*, **2018**, *7*(1), 76-84.
[PMID: 30324121]

[3]   Parthiban, K.G.; Kumar, B.S.; Kumar, R.M.N.S. Herbal drug comprehensive approach for treating liver disease and focus towards herbal medicine. *Int. J. Curr. Res. Rev.*, **2010**, *2*(3), 3-15.

[4]   Pandey, S.; Darunde, D. Herbal drugs :An approach for the treatment of liver disorders. *International Journal of Pharmacognosy,* **2019**, *6*(5), 164-171.

[5]   Wagner, H.; Wolff, P.M. New natural products and plant drugs with pharmacological, biological or therapeutic activity. *Proceedings of the First International Congress on Medicinal Plant Research, Section A, Held at the University of Munich,* GermanySeptember 6–10, 1976**2012**.

[6]   Licata, A.; Macaluso, F.S.; Craxì, A. Herbal hepatotoxicity: A hidden epidemic. *Intern. Emerg. Med.,* **2013**, *8*(1), 13-22.
[http://dx.doi.org/10.1007/s11739-012-0777-x] [PMID: 22477279]

[7]   Ali, SA; Sharief, NH; Mohamed, YS *Hepatoprotective activity of some medicinal plants in Sudan., Evid Based Complement Alternat Med.,* **2019**, *2019*, 2196315.
[http://dx.doi.org/10.1155/2019/2196315]

[8]   Panda, A.; Bhuyan, G.; Rao, M. Ayurvedic intervention for hepatobiliary disorders: Current scenario and future prospect. *J Tradit Med Clin Natur.,* **2017**, *6*(210), 2.

[9]   Hasan, M.A. A review on hepatoprotective activity of various medicinal plant. *Faslnamah-i Giyahan-i Daruyi,* **2020**, *8*(5), 204-207.

[10]   Meng, X.; Li, Y.; Li, S.; Gan, R.Y.; Li, H.B. Natural products for prevention and treatment of chemical-induced liver injuries. *Compr. Rev. Food Sci. Food Saf.,* **2018**, *17*(2), 472-495. [http://dx.doi.org/10.1111/1541-4337.12335] [PMID: 33350084]

[11]   Srivastava, R.; Srivastava, P. Hepatotoxicity and the role of some herbal hepatoprotective plants in present scenario. *I. J. Diges.Dis.,* **2018**, *4*(2), 2. [http://dx.doi.org/10.4172/2472-1891.100034]

[12]   Alhassan, A.J.; Lawal, T.A.; Dangambo, M. Antidiabetic properties of thirteen local medicinal plants in nigeria, a review. *World J. Pharm. Res.,* **2017**, *6523*(8), 2170-2189. [http://dx.doi.org/10.20959/wjpr20178-9055]

[13]   Kulkarni, K.V.; Adavirao, B.V. A review on: Indian traditional shrub Tulsi (*Ocimum sanctum*): The unique medicinal plant. *Journal of Medicinal Plants Studies.,* **2018**, *6*(2), 106-110.

[14]   Bano, N.; Ahmed, A.; Tanveer, M.; Khan, G.; Ansari, M. Pharmacological evaluation of Ocimum sanctum. *J. Bioequivalence Bioavailab.,* **2017**, *9*(3), 387-392.

[15]   Sadashiva, C.; Hussain, H.F.; Nanjundaiah, S. Evaluation of hepatoprotective, antioxidant and cytotoxic properties of aqueous extract of turmeric rhizome (Turmesac). *J. Med. Plants Res.,* **2019**, *13*(17), 423-430.

[16]   Douichene, S.; Rached, W.; Djebli, N. Hepato-protective effect of curcuma longa against paracetamol-induced chronic hepatotoxicity in swiss mice. *Jordan J. Biol. Sci.,* **2020**, *13*(3), 275-279.

[17]   Lukitaningsih, E. *In vivo* antioxidant activities of curcuma longa and curcuma xanthorrhiza. *Food Res.,* **2020**, *4*(1), 13-19. [http://dx.doi.org/10.26656/fr.2017.4(1).172]

[18]   Salama, S.M.; Abdulla, M.A.; AlRashdi, A.S.; Ismail, S.; Alkiyumi, S.S.; Golbabapour, S. Hepatoprotective effect of ethanolic extract of Curcuma longa on thioacetamide induced liver cirrhosis in rats. *BMC Complement. Altern. Med.,* **2013**, *13*(1), 56. [http://dx.doi.org/10.1186/1472-6882-13-56] [PMID: 23496995]

[19]   Ramirez-Boscá, A.; Soler, A.; Carrión Gutierrez, M.A.; Laborda Alvarez, J.; Quintanilla Almagro, E. Antioxidant curcuma extracts decrease the blood lipid peroxide levels of human subjects. *Age,* **1995**, *18*(4), 167-169. [http://dx.doi.org/10.1007/BF02432631]

[20]   Satoskar, R.R.; Shah, S.J.; Shenoy, S.G. Evaluation of anti-inflammatory property of curcumin (diferuloyl methane) in patients with postoperative inflammation. *Int. J. Clin. Pharmacol. Ther. Toxicol.,* **1986**, *24*(12), 651-654. [PMID: 3546166]

[21]   Shankar, T.N.; Shantha, N.V.; Ramesh, H.P.; Murthy, I.A.; Murthy, V.S. Toxicity studies on turmeric (Curcuma longa): acute toxicity studies in rats, guineapigs & monkeys. *Indian J. Exp. Biol.,* **1980**, *18*(1), 73-75. [PMID: 6772551]

[22]   Tripathi, UN; Chandra, D Hepatoprotective potential of trigonella foenum graecum in deltamethrin induced albino rats. *Indian Journal of Pharmaceutical and Biological Research.,* **2014**, *2*(04), 1-8. [http://dx.doi.org/10.30750/ijpbr.2.4.1]

[23]   Das, S. Hepatoprotective activity of methanol extract of fenugreek seeds on rats. *Int. J. Pharm. Sci. Res.,* **2014**, *5*(4), 1506.

[24]   Zargar, S. Protective effect of *Trigonella foenum-graecum* on thioacetamide induced hepatotoxicity in rats. *Saudi J. Biol. Sci.,* **2014**, *21*(2), 139-145. [http://dx.doi.org/10.1016/j.sjbs.2013.09.002] [PMID: 24600306]

[25]   Habib, M.; Waheed, I. Evaluation of anti-nociceptive, anti-inflammatory and antipyretic activities of Artemisia scoparia hydromethanolic extract. *J. Ethnopharmacol.,* **2013**, *145*(1), 18-24.

[http://dx.doi.org/10.1016/j.jep.2012.10.022] [PMID: 23117091]

[26]   Singh, H.; Mittal, S.; Kaur, S.; Batish, D.; Kohli, R. Chemical composition and antioxidant activity of essential oil from residues of artemisia scoparia. *Food Chem.,* **2009**, *114*(2), 642-645.
[http://dx.doi.org/10.1016/j.foodchem.2008.09.101]

[27]   Ali, B.H.; Bashir, A.K.; Rasheed, R.A. Effect of the traditional medicinal plants rhazya stricta, balanitis aegyptiaca and haplophylum tuberculatum on paracetamol-induced hepatotoxicity in mice. *Phytother. Res.,* **2001**, *15*(7), 598-603.
[http://dx.doi.org/10.1002/ptr.818] [PMID: 11746841]

[28]   Jaiprakash, B.; Karadi, R.; Savadi, R.; Hukkeri, V. Hepatoprotective activity of bark of balanites aegyptiaca linn. *J. Nat. Rem.,* **2003**, *3*(2), 205-207.

[29]   Obidah, W.; Nadro, M.S.; Tiyafo, G.O.; Wurochekke, A.U. Toxicity of crude Balanites aegyptiaca seed oil in rats. *J. Am. Sci.,* **2009**, *5*(6), 13-16.

[30]   Popović, M.; Kaurinović, B.; Trivić, S.; Mimica-Dukić, N.; Bursać, M. Effect of celery (apium graveolens) extracts on some biochemical parameters of oxidative stress in mice treated with carbon tetrachloride. *Phytother. Res.,* **2006**, *20*(7), 531-537.
[http://dx.doi.org/10.1002/ptr.1871] [PMID: 16685681]

[31]   Menon, B.R.; Rathi, M.A.; Thirumoorthi, L.; Gopalakrishnan, V.K. Potential effect of bacopa monnieri on nitrobenzene induced liver damage in rats. *Indian J. Clin. Biochem.,* **2010**, *25*(4), 401-404.
[http://dx.doi.org/10.1007/s12291-010-0048-4] [PMID: 21966114]

[32]   Sumathy, T.; Govindasamy, S.; Balakrishna, K.; Veluchamy, G. Protective role of Bacopa monniera on morphine-induced brain mitochondrial enzyme activity in rats. *Fitoterapia,* **2002**, *73*(5), 381-385.
[http://dx.doi.org/10.1016/S0367-326X(02)00114-4] [PMID: 12165332]

[33]   Joshua Allan, J.; Damodaran, A.; Deshmukh, N.S.; Goudar, K.S.; Amit, A. Safety evaluation of a standardized phytochemical composition extracted from bacopa monnieri in sprague–dawley rats. *Food Chem. Toxicol.,* **2007**, *45*(10), 1928-1937.
[http://dx.doi.org/10.1016/j.fct.2007.04.010] [PMID: 17560704]

[34]   Agarwal, M.; Srivastava, V.K.; Saxena, K.K.; Kumar, A. Hepatoprotective activity of beta vulgaris against ccl4-induced hepatic injury in rats. *Fitoterapia,* **2006**, *77*(2), 91-93.
[http://dx.doi.org/10.1016/j.fitote.2005.11.004] [PMID: 16376022]

[35]   Georgiev, V.G.; Weber, J.; Kneschke, E.M.; Denev, P.N.; Bley, T.; Pavlov, A.I. Antioxidant activity and phenolic content of betalain extracts from intact plants and hairy root cultures of the red beetroot Beta vulgaris cv. Detroit dark red. *Plant Foods Hum. Nutr.,* **2010**, *65*(2), 105-111.
[http://dx.doi.org/10.1007/s11130-010-0156-6] [PMID: 20195764]

[36]   Sengottuvelu, S.; Duraisami, S.; Nandhakumar, J.; Duraisami, R.; Vasudevan, M. Hepatoprotective activity of Camellia sinensis and its possible mechanism of action. *Iranian Journal of Pharmacology and Therapeutics,* **2008**, *7*(1), 9-14.

[37]   Al-Asmari, A.K.; Al-Elaiwi, A.M.; Athar, M.T.; Tariq, M.; Al Eid, A.; Al-Asmary, S.M. A review of hepatoprotective plants used in saudi traditional medicine. *Evid. Based Complement. Alternat. Med.,* **2014**, *2014*, 1-22.
[http://dx.doi.org/10.1155/2014/890842] [PMID: 25587347]

[38]   Olaleye, M.T.; Akinmoladun, A.C.; Ogunboye, A.A.; Akindahunsi, A.A. Antioxidant activity and hepatoprotective property of leaf extracts of Boerhaavia diffusa Linn against acetaminophen-induced liver damage in rats. *Food Chem. Toxicol.,* **2010**, *48*(8-9), 2200-2205.
[http://dx.doi.org/10.1016/j.fct.2010.05.047] [PMID: 20553784]

[39]   Devaki, T.; Shivashangari, K.; Ravikumar, V.; Govindaraju, P. Hepatoprotective activity of Boerhaavia diffusa on ethanol-induced liver damage in rats. *J. Nat. Rem.,* **2004**, *4*(2), 109-115.

[40]   Orisakwe, O.E.; Afonne, O.J.; Chude, M.A.; Obi, E.; Dioka, C.E. Sub-chronic toxicity studies of the

aqueous extract of Boerhavia diffusa leaves. *J. Health Sci.,* **2003**, *49*(6), 444-447.
[http://dx.doi.org/10.1248/jhs.49.444]

[41] Schuppan, D.; Jia, J.D.; Brinkhaus, B.; Hahn, E.G. Herbal products for liver diseases: A therapeutic challenge for the new millennium. *Hepatology,* **1999**, *30*(4), 1099-1104.
[http://dx.doi.org/10.1002/hep.510300437] [PMID: 10498665]

[42] Singab, A.N.B.; Ayoub, N.A.; Ali, E.N.; Mostafa, N.M. Antioxidant and hepatoprotective activities of Egyptian moraceous plants against carbon tetrachloride-induced oxidative stress and liver damage in rats. *Pharm. Biol.,* **2010**, *48*(11), 1255-1264.
[http://dx.doi.org/10.3109/13880201003730659] [PMID: 20839909]

[43] Gond, N.Y.; Khadabadi, S.S. Hepatoprotective activity of <i> Ficus carica</i> leaf extract on rifampicin-induced hepatic damage in rats. *Indian J. Pharm. Sci.,* **2008**, *70*(3), 364-366.
[http://dx.doi.org/10.4103/0250-474X.43003] [PMID: 20046747]

[44] Bonamonte, D.; Foti, C.; Lionetti, N.; Rigano, L.; Angelini, G. Photoallergic contact dermatitis to 8-methoxypsoralen in Ficus carica. *Contact Dermat.,* **2010**, *62*(6), 343-348.
[http://dx.doi.org/10.1111/j.1600-0536.2010.01713.x] [PMID: 20557340]

[45] Safa, O.; Soltanipoor, M.A.; Rastegar, S.; Kazemi, M.; Nourbakhsh Dehkordi, K.; Ghannadi, A. An ethnobotanical survey on hormozgan province, Iran. *Avicenna J. Phytomed.,* **2013**, *3*(1), 64-81.
[PMID: 25050260]

[46] Al-Said, M.S.; Mothana, R.A.; Al-Sohaibani, M.O.; Rafatullah, S. Ameliorative effect of Grewia tenax (Forssk) fiori fruit extract on CCl(4)-induced oxidative stress and hepatotoxicity in rats. *J. Food Sci.,* **2011**, *76*(9), T200-T206.
[http://dx.doi.org/10.1111/j.1750-3841.2011.02381.x] [PMID: 22416728]

[47] Alqasoumi, S. Carbon tetrachloride-induced hepatotoxicity: Protective effect of 'Rocket' Eruca sativa L. in rats. *Am. J. Chin. Med.,* **2010**, *38*(1), 75-88.
[http://dx.doi.org/10.1142/S0192415X10007671] [PMID: 20128046]

[48] Hussein, J.; Salah, A.; Oraby, F.; El-Deen, A.N.; El-Khayat, Z. Antihepatotoxic effect of Eruca sativa extracts on alcohol induced liver injury in rats. *J. Am. Sci.,* **2010**, *6*(11), 381-389.

[49] Asuku, O.; Atawodi, S.E.; Onyike, E. Antioxidant, hepatoprotective, and ameliorative effects of methanolic extract of leaves of Grewia mollis Juss. on carbon tetrachloride-treated albino rats. *J. Med. Food,* **2012**, *15*(1), 83-88.
[http://dx.doi.org/10.1089/jmf.2010.0285] [PMID: 21877945]

[50] Obidah, W.; Godwin, J.L.; Fate, J.Z.; Madusolumuo, M.A. Toxic effects of grewia mollis stem bark in experimental rats. *J. Am. Sci.,* **2010**, *6*(12), 1544-1548.

[51] Abuelgasim, A.I.; Nuha, H.; Mohammed, A. Hepatoprotective effect of Lepidium sativum against carbon tetrachloride induced damage in rats. *Res J.Ani.and Veterinary Sciences.,* **2008**, *3*, 20-23.

[52] Adam, S. Effects of various levels of dietary Lepidium sativum L. seeds in rats. *The American journal of Chinese medicine.,* **1999**, *27*(03n04), 397-405.

[53] Rivera-Espinoza, Y.; Muriel, P. Pharmacological actions of curcumin in liver diseases or damage. *Liver Int.,* **2009**, *29*(10), 1457-1466.
[http://dx.doi.org/10.1111/j.1478-3231.2009.02086.x] [PMID: 19811613]

[54] Polyak, S.J.; Morishima, C.; Lohmann, V.; Pal, S.; Lee, D.Y.W.; Liu, Y.; Graf, T.N.; Oberlies, N.H. Identification of hepatoprotective flavonolignans from silymarin. *Proc. Natl. Acad. Sci.,* **2010**, *107*(13), 5995-5999.
[http://dx.doi.org/10.1073/pnas.0914009107] [PMID: 20231449]

[55] Chirdchupunseree, H.; Pramyothin, P. Protective activity of phyllanthin in ethanol-treated primary culture of rat hepatocytes. *J. Ethnopharmacol.,* **2010**, *128*(1), 172-176.
[http://dx.doi.org/10.1016/j.jep.2010.01.003] [PMID: 20064596]

[56]   Wan, X.; Luo, M.; Li, X.; He, P. Hepatoprotective and anti-hepatocarcinogenic effects of glycyrrhizin and matrine. *Chem. Biol. Interact.,* **2009**, *181*(1), 15-19.
[http://dx.doi.org/10.1016/j.cbi.2009.04.013] [PMID: 19426721]

[57]   Rathore, P.; Rao, S.P.; Roy, A.; Satapathy, T.; Singh, V.; Jain, P. Hepatoprotective activity of isolated herbal compounds. *Research Journal of Pharmacy and Technology.,* **2014**, *7*(2), 229-234.

[58]   Rao, G.M.M.; Rao, C.V.; Pushpangadan, P.; Shirwaikar, A. Hepatoprotective effects of rubiadin, a major constituent of Rubia cordifolia Linn. *J. Ethnopharmacol.,* **2006**, *103*(3), 484-490.
[http://dx.doi.org/10.1016/j.jep.2005.08.073] [PMID: 16213120]

[59]   Banskota, A.H.; Tezuka, Y.; Adnyana, I.K.; Ishii, E.; Midorikawa, K.; Matsushige, K.; Kadota, S. Hepatoprotective and anti-Helicobacter pylori activities of constituents from Brazilian propolis. *Phytomedicine,* **2001**, *8*(1), 16-23.
[http://dx.doi.org/10.1078/0944-7113-00004] [PMID: 11292234]

[60]   Nithianantham, K.; Ping, K.Y.; Latha, L.Y.; Jothy, S.L.; Darah, I.; Chen, Y.; Chew, A.L.; Sasidharan, S. Evaluation of hepatoprotective effect of methanolic extract of Clitoria ternatea (Linn.) flower against acetaminophen-induced liver damage. *Asian Pac. J. Trop. Dis.,* **2013**, *3*(4), 314-319.
[http://dx.doi.org/10.1016/S2222-1808(13)60075-4]

[61]   Sánchez-Salgado, J.C.; Ortiz-Andrade, R.R.; Aguirre-Crespo, F.; Vergara-Galicia, J.; León-Rivera, I.; Montes, S.; Villalobos-Molina, R.; Estrada-Soto, S. Hypoglycemic, vasorelaxant and hepatoprotective effects of *Cochlospermum vitifolium (Willd.) Sprengel* : A potential agent for the treatment of metabolic syndrome. *J. Ethnopharmacol.,* **2007**, *109*(3), 400-405.
[http://dx.doi.org/10.1016/j.jep.2006.08.008] [PMID: 16978815]

[62]   Awaad, A.S.; Maitland, D.J.; Soliman, G.A. Hepatoprotective activity of schouwia thebica webb. *Bioorg. Med. Chem. Lett.,* **2006**, *16*(17), 4624-4628.
[http://dx.doi.org/10.1016/j.bmcl.2006.06.011] [PMID: 16797983]

[63]   Hong, Z.; Chen, W.; Zhao, J.; Wu, Z.; Zhou, J.; Li, T.; Hu, J. Hepatoprotective effects of Rubus aleaefolius Poir. and identification of its active constituents. *J. Ethnopharmacol.,* **2010**, *129*(2), 267-272.
[http://dx.doi.org/10.1016/j.jep.2010.03.025] [PMID: 20362654]

[64]   Adebajo, A.C.; Iwalewa, E.O.; Obuotor, E.M.; Ibikunle, G.F.; Omisore, N.O.; Adewunmi, C.O.; Obaparusi, O.O.; Klaes, M.; Adetogun, G.E.; Schmidt, T.J.; Verspohl, E.J. Pharmacological properties of the extract and some isolated compounds of Clausena lansium stem bark: Anti-trichomonal, antidiabetic, anti-inflammatory, hepatoprotective and antioxidant effects. *J. Ethnopharmacol.,* **2009**, *122*(1), 10-19.
[http://dx.doi.org/10.1016/j.jep.2008.11.015] [PMID: 19095054]

[65]   Sabir, S.M.; Rocha, J.B.T. Antioxidant and hepatoprotective activity of aqueous extract of Solanum fastigiatum (false "Jurubeba") against paracetamol-induced liver damage in mice. *J. Ethnopharmacol.,* **2008**, *120*(2), 226-232.
[http://dx.doi.org/10.1016/j.jep.2008.08.017] [PMID: 18790038]

[66]   Karthikeyan, R.; Somasundaram, S.T.; Manivasagam, T.; Balasubramanian, T.; Anantharaman, P. Hepatoprotective activity of brown alga Padina boergesenii against CCl4 induced oxidative damage in wistar rats. *Asian Pac. J. Trop. Med.,* **2010**, *3*(9), 696-701.
[http://dx.doi.org/10.1016/S1995-7645(10)60168-X]

[67]   Jain, N.K.; Singhai, A.K. Protective effects of phyllanthus acidus (l.) skeels leaf extracts on acetaminophen and thioacetamide induced hepatic injuries in wistar rats. *Asian Pac. J. Trop. Med.,* **2011**, *4*(6), 470-474.
[http://dx.doi.org/10.1016/S1995-7645(11)60128-4] [PMID: 21771701]

[68]   Noh, J.R.; Kim, Y.H.; Gang, G.T.; Hwang, J.H.; Lee, H.S.; Ly, S.Y.; Oh, W.K.; Song, K.S.; Lee, C.H. Hepatoprotective effects of chestnut (Castanea crenata) inner shell extract against chronic ethanol-induced oxidative stress in C57BL/6 mice. *Food Chem. Toxicol.,* **2011**, *49*(7), 1537-1543.

[http://dx.doi.org/10.1016/j.fct.2011.03.045] [PMID: 21457746]

[69]   Huang, Q.; Zhang, S.; Huang, R.; Wei, L.; Chen, Y.; Lv, S.; Liang, C.; Tan, S.; liang, S.; Zhuo, L.; Lin, X. Isolation and identification of an anti-hepatitis B virus compound from Hydrocotyle sibthorpioides Lam. *J. Ethnopharmacol.,* **2013**, *150*(2), 568-575. [http://dx.doi.org/10.1016/j.jep.2013.09.009] [PMID: 24051027]

[70]   Rao, K.S.; Mishra, S.H. Antihepatotoxic activity of monomethyl fumarate isolated from *Fumaria indica* . *J. Ethnopharmacol.,* **1998**, *60*(3), 207-213. [http://dx.doi.org/10.1016/S0378-8741(97)00149-9] [PMID: 9613834]

[71]   Ao, Z.H.; Xu, Z.H.; Lu, Z.M.; Xu, H.Y.; Zhang, X.M.; Dou, W.F. Niuchangchih (Antrodia camphorata) and its potential in treating liver diseases. *J. Ethnopharmacol.,* **2009**, *121*(2), 194-212. [http://dx.doi.org/10.1016/j.jep.2008.10.039] [PMID: 19061947]

[72]   Vicente, G.; Molina, S.; González-Vallinas, M.; García-Risco, M.R.; Fornari, T.; Reglero, G.; de Molina, A.R. Supercritical rosemary extracts, their antioxidant activity and effect on hepatic tumor progression. *J. Supercrit. Fluids,* **2013**, *79*, 101-108. [http://dx.doi.org/10.1016/j.supflu.2012.07.006]

[73]   Arun, M.; Asha, V.V. Preliminary studies on antihepatotoxic effect of Physalis peruviana Linn. (Solanaceae) against carbon tetrachloride induced acute liver injury in rats. *J. Ethnopharmacol.,* **2007**, *111*(1), 110-114. [http://dx.doi.org/10.1016/j.jep.2006.10.038] [PMID: 17161567]

[74]   El Denshary, E.S.; Al-Gahazali, M.A.; Mannaa, F.A.; Salem, H.A.; Hassan, N.S.; Abdel-Wahhab, M.A. Dietary honey and ginseng protect against carbon tetrachloride-induced hepatonephrotoxicity in rats. *Exp. Toxicol. Pathol.,* **2012**, *64*(7-8), 753-760. [http://dx.doi.org/10.1016/j.etp.2011.01.012] [PMID: 21330121]

[75]   Lee, M.K.; Ha, N.R.; Yang, H.; Sung, S.H.; Kim, G.H.; Kim, Y.C. Antiproliferative activity of triterpenoids from Eclipta prostrata on hepatic stellate cells. *Phytomedicine,* **2008**, *15*(9), 775-780. [http://dx.doi.org/10.1016/j.phymed.2007.10.004] [PMID: 18061418]

[76]   Ko, J.H.; Lee, S.J.; Lim, K.T. Rhus verniciflua Stokes glycoprotein (36kDa) has protective activity on carbon tetrachloride-induced liver injury in mice. *Environ. Toxicol. Pharmacol.,* **2006**, *22*(1), 8-14. [http://dx.doi.org/10.1016/j.etap.2005.10.005] [PMID: 21783679]

[77]   Sunitha, S.; Nagaraj, M.; Varalakshmi, P. Hepatoprotective effect of lupeol and lupeol linoleate on tissue antioxidant defence system in cadmium-induced hepatotoxicity in rats. *Fitoterapia,* **2001**, *72*(5), 516-523. [http://dx.doi.org/10.1016/S0367-326X(01)00259-3] [PMID: 11429246]

[78]   Benedek, B.; Geisz, N.; Jäger, W.; Thalhammer, T.; Kopp, B. Choleretic effects of yarrow (Achillea millefolium s.l.) in the isolated perfused rat liver. *Phytomedicine,* **2006**, *13*(9-10), 702-706. [http://dx.doi.org/10.1016/j.phymed.2005.10.005] [PMID: 16303291]

[79]   Jain, A.; Soni, M.; Deb, L.; Jain, A.; Rout, S.P.; Gupta, V.B.; Krishna, K.L. Antioxidant and hepatoprotective activity of ethanolic and aqueous extracts of Momordica dioica Roxb. leaves. *J. Ethnopharmacol.,* **2008**, *115*(1), 61-66. [http://dx.doi.org/10.1016/j.jep.2007.09.009] [PMID: 17983713]

[80]   Kamat, J.P.; Boloor, K.K.; Devasagayam, T.P.A.; Venkatachalam, S.R. Antioxidant properties of Asparagus racemosus against damage induced by γ-radiation in rat liver mitochondria. *J. Ethnopharmacol.,* **2000**, *71*(3), 425-435. [http://dx.doi.org/10.1016/S0378-8741(00)00176-8] [PMID: 10940579]

[81]   Ahmed, B.; Alam, T.; Khan, S.A. Hepatoprotective activity of Luffa echinata fruits. *J. Ethnopharmacol.,* **2001**, *76*(2), 187-189. [http://dx.doi.org/10.1016/S0378-8741(00)00402-5] [PMID: 11390135]

[82]   Chandan, B.K.; Saxena, A.K.; Shukla, S.; Sharma, N.; Gupta, D.K.; Suri, K.A.; Suri, J.; Bhadauria,

M.; Singh, B. Hepatoprotective potential of Aloe barbadensis Mill. against carbon tetrachloride induced hepatotoxicity. *J. Ethnopharmacol.,* **2007**, *111*(3), 560-566.
[http://dx.doi.org/10.1016/j.jep.2007.01.008] [PMID: 17291700]

[83]   Dhanasekaran, M.; Ignacimuthu, S.; Agastian, P. Potential hepatoprotective activity of ononitol monohydrate isolated from Cassia tora L. on carbon tetrachloride induced hepatotoxicity in wistar rats. *Phytomedicine,* **2009**, *16*(9), 891-895.
[http://dx.doi.org/10.1016/j.phymed.2009.02.006] [PMID: 19345078]

[84]   Jayasekhar, P.; Mohanan, P.; Rathinam, K. Hepatoprotective activity of ethyl acetate extract of Acacia catechu. *Indian J. Pharmacol.,* **1997**, *29*(6), 426.

[85]   Gujrati, V.; Patel, N.; Rao, V.N. Hepatoprotective activity of alcoholic and aqueous extracts of leaves of Tylophora indica (Linn.) in rats. *Indian J. Pharmacol.,* **2007**, *39*(1), 43.
[http://dx.doi.org/10.4103/0253-7613.30763]

[86]   Kumar, C.H.; Ramesh, A.; Kumar, J.S.; Ishaq, B.M. A review on hepatoprotective activity of medicinal plants. *Int. J. Pharm. Sci. Res.,* **2011**, *2*(3), 501.

[87]   Tung, Y.T.; Wu, J.H.; Huang, C.C.; Peng, H.C.; Chen, Y.L.; Yang, S.C.; Chang, S.T. Protective effect of Acacia confusa bark extract and its active compound gallic acid against carbon tetrachloride-induced chronic liver injury in rats. *Food Chem. Toxicol.,* **2009**, *47*(6), 1385-1392.
[http://dx.doi.org/10.1016/j.fct.2009.03.021] [PMID: 19327382]

[88]   Gilani, A.H.; Jabeen, Q.; Ghayur, M.N.; Janbaz, K.H.; Akhtar, M.S. Studies on the antihypertensive, antispasmodic, bronchodilator and hepatoprotective activities of the Carum copticum seed extract. *J. Ethnopharmacol.,* **2005**, *98*(1-2), 127-135.
[http://dx.doi.org/10.1016/j.jep.2005.01.017] [PMID: 15763373]

[89]   Wang, N.; Li, P.; Wang, Y.; Peng, W.; Wu, Z.; Tan, S.; Liang, S.; Shen, X.; Su, W. Hepatoprotective effect of Hypericum japonicum extract and its fractions. *J. Ethnopharmacol.,* **2008**, *116*(1), 1-6.
[http://dx.doi.org/10.1016/j.jep.2007.08.031] [PMID: 18178045]

[90]   Anusuya, N.; Raju, K.; Manian, S. Hepatoprotective and toxicological assessment of an ethnomedicinal plant Euphorbia fusiformis Buch.-Ham.ex D.Don. *J. Ethnopharmacol.,* **2010**, *127*(2), 463-467.
[http://dx.doi.org/10.1016/j.jep.2009.10.012] [PMID: 19837150]

[91]   Wang, B.J.; Liu, C.T.; Tseng, C.Y.; Wu, C.P.; Yu, Z.R. Hepatoprotective and antioxidant effects of Bupleurum kaoi Liu (Chao et Chuang) extract and its fractions fractionated using supercritical CO2 on CCl4-induced liver damage. *Food Chem. Toxicol.,* **2004**, *42*(4), 609-617.
[http://dx.doi.org/10.1016/j.fct.2003.11.011] [PMID: 15019185]

[92]   Wu, Y.; Yang, L.; Wang, F.; Wu, X.; Zhou, C.; Shi, S.; Mo, J.; Zhao, Y. Hepatoprotective and antioxidative effects of total phenolics from Laggera pterodonta on chemical-induced injury in primary cultured neonatal rat hepatocytes. *Food Chem. Toxicol.,* **2007**, *45*(8), 1349-1355.
[http://dx.doi.org/10.1016/j.fct.2007.01.011] [PMID: 17329003]

[93]   Aqil, F.; Munagala, R.; Jeyabalan, J.; Vadhanam, M.V. Bioavailability of phytochemicals and its enhancement by drug delivery systems. *Cancer Lett.,* **2013**, *334*(1), 133-141.
[http://dx.doi.org/10.1016/j.canlet.2013.02.032] [PMID: 23435377]

[94]   Adhami, V.M.; Mukhtar, H. Human cancer chemoprevention: Hurdles and challenges. *Top. Curr. Chem.,* **2012**, *329*, 203-220.
[http://dx.doi.org/10.1007/128_2012_342] [PMID: 22790416]

[95]   Bharali, D.J.; Siddiqui, I.A.; Adhami, V.M.; Chamcheu, J.C.; Aldahmash, A.M.; Mukhtar, H.; Mousa, S.A. Nanoparticle delivery of natural products in the prevention and treatment of cancers: Current status and future prospects. *Cancers,* **2011**, *3*(4), 4024-4045.
[http://dx.doi.org/10.3390/cancers3044024] [PMID: 24213123]

[96]   Wang, S.; Su, R.; Nie, S.; Sun, M.; Zhang, J.; Wu, D.; Moustaid-Moussa, N. Application of

nanotechnology in improving bioavailability and bioactivity of diet-derived phytochemicals. *J. Nutr. Biochem.,* **2014**, *25*(4), 363-376.
[http://dx.doi.org/10.1016/j.jnutbio.2013.10.002] [PMID: 24406273]

[97] Din, F.; Aman, W.; Ullah, I.; Qureshi, O.S.; Mustapha, O.; Shafique, S.; Zeb, A. Effective use of nanocarriers as drug delivery systems for the treatment of selected tumors. *Int. J. Nanomedicine,* **2017**, *12*, 7291-7309.
[http://dx.doi.org/10.2147/IJN.S146315] [PMID: 29042776]

[98] Kassem, A.A.; Abd El-Alim, S.H.; Salman, A.M.; Mohammed, M.A.; Hassan, N.S.; El-Gengaihi, S.E. Improved hepatoprotective activity of *Beta vulgaris* L. leaf extract loaded self-nanoemulsifying drug delivery system (SNEDDS): *in vitro* and *in vivo* evaluation. *Drug Dev. Ind. Pharm.,* **2020**, *46*(10), 1589-1603.
[http://dx.doi.org/10.1080/03639045.2020.1811303] [PMID: 32811211]

[99] Yen, F.L.; Wu, T.H.; Lin, L.T.; Cham, T.M.; Lin, C.C. Nanoparticles formulation of *Cuscuta chinensis* prevents acetaminophen-induced hepatotoxicity in rats. *Food Chem. Toxicol.,* **2008**, *46*(5), 1771-1777.
[http://dx.doi.org/10.1016/j.fct.2008.01.021] [PMID: 18308443]

[100] Deepa, V.; Sridhar, R.; Goparaju, A.; Reddy, P.N.; Murthy, P.B. Nanoemulsified ethanolic extract of *Pyllanthus amarus* Schum & *Thonn ameliorates* CCl_4 induced hepatotoxicity in Wistar rats. *Indian J. Exp. Biol.,* **2012**, *50*(11), 785-794.
[PMID: 23305029]

[101] Aisha, A.F.A.; Majid, A.M.S.A.; Ismail, Z. Preparation and characterization of nano liposomes of *Orthosiphon stamineus*ethanolic extract in soybean phospholipids. *BMC Biotechnol.,* **2014**, *14*(1), 23.
[http://dx.doi.org/10.1186/1472-6750-14-23] [PMID: 24674107]

[102] Maiti, K.; Mukherjee, K.; Murugan, V.; Saha, B.P.; Mukherjee, P.K. Enhancing bioavailability and hepatoprotective activity of andrographolide from *Andrographis paniculata*, a well-known medicinal food, through its herbosome. *J. Sci. Food Agric.,* **2010**, *90*(1), 43-51.
[http://dx.doi.org/10.1002/jsfa.3777] [PMID: 20355010]

[103] Abdou, E.M.; Fayed, M.A.A.; Helal, D.; Ahmed, K.A. Assessment of the hepatoprotective effect of developed lipid-polymer hybrid nanoparticles (LPHNPs) encapsulating naturally extracted β-Sitosterol against CCl_4 induced hepatotoxicity in rats. *Sci. Rep.,* **2019**, *9*(1), 19779.
[http://dx.doi.org/10.1038/s41598-019-56320-2] [PMID: 31875004]

[104] Prakash, E.; Jeyadoss, T.; Velavan, S. *In vitro* hepatoprotective activity of Azima tetracantha leaf extract and silver nanoparticle in hepatocytes. *Pharma Chem.,* **2015**, *7*(10), 381-390.

[105] Zhang, H.; Jacob, J.A.; Jiang, Z.; Xu, S.; Sun, K.; Zhong, Z.; Varadharaju, N.; Shanmugam, A. Hepatoprotective effect of silver nanoparticles synthesized using aqueous leaf extract of *Rhizophora apiculata*. *Int. J. Nanomedicine,* **2019**, *14*, 3517-3524.
[http://dx.doi.org/10.2147/IJN.S198895] [PMID: 31190808]

[106] Yang, K.Y.; Hwang, H.; Yousaf, A.M.; Kim, D.W.; Shin, Y.J.; Bae, O.N.; Kim, Y.I.; Kim, J.O.; Yong, C.S.; Choi, H.G. Silymarin-loaded solid nanoparticles provide excellent hepatic protection: Physicochemical characterization and in vivo evaluation. *Int. J. Nanomedicine,* **2013**, *8*, 3333-3343.
[PMID: 24039417]

[107] Maheshwari, H.; Agarwal, R.; Patil, C.; Katare, O.P. Preparation and pharmacological evaluation of silibinin liposomes. *Arzneimittelforschung,* **2003**, *53*(6), 420-427.
[PMID: 12872613]

[108] Seeff, L.B. Herbal Hepatotoxicity. *Clin. Liver Dis.,* **2007**, *11*(3), 577-596, vii.
[http://dx.doi.org/10.1016/j.cld.2007.06.005] [PMID: 17723921]

[109] Daniele, C.; Dahamna, S.; Firuzi, O.; Sekfali, N.; Saso, L.; Mazzanti, G. Atractylis gummifera L. poisoning: An ethnopharmacological review. *J. Ethnopharmacol.,* **2005**, *97*(2), 175-181.
[http://dx.doi.org/10.1016/j.jep.2004.11.025] [PMID: 15707749]

[110] Bouziri, A.; Hamdi, A.; Menif, K.; Ben Jaballah, N. Hepatorenal injury induced by cutaneous application of *Atractylis gummifera* L. *Clin. Toxicol.,* **2010**, *48*(7), 752-754.
[http://dx.doi.org/10.3109/15563650.2010.498379] [PMID: 20615152]

[111] HAMOUDA, C. A review of acute poisoning from Atractylis gummifera L. *Journal of Emergency Actors.,* **2004**, *3*, 23-26.

[112] Steenkamp, P.; Harding, N.; Heerden, F.; Wyk, B. Determination of atractyloside in Callilepis laureola using solid-phase extraction and liquid chromatography–atmospheric pressure ionisation mass spectrometry. *J. Chromatogr. A,* **2004**, *1058*(1-2), 153-162.
[http://dx.doi.org/10.1016/S0021-9673(04)01305-6] [PMID: 15595663]

[113] Popat, A.; Shear, N.H.; Malkiewicz, I.; Stewart, M.J.; Steenkamp, V.; Thomson, S.; Neuman, M.G. The toxicity of callilepis laureola, a south african traditional herbal medicine. *Clin. Biochem.,* **2001**, *34*(3), 229-236.
[http://dx.doi.org/10.1016/S0009-9120(01)00219-3] [PMID: 11408021]

[114] Popat, A.; Shear, N.H.; Malkiewicz, I.; Thomson, S.; Neuman, M.G. Mechanism of *Impila (Callilepis laureola)* :Induced cytotoxicity in Hep G2 cells. *Clin. Biochem.,* **2002**, *35*(1), 57-64.
[http://dx.doi.org/10.1016/S0009-9120(02)00271-0] [PMID: 11937079]

[115] Kassler, W.J.; Blanc, P.; Greenblatt, R. The use of medicinal herbs by human immunodeficiency virus-infected patients. *Arch. Intern. Med.,* **1991**, *151*(11), 2281-2288.
[http://dx.doi.org/10.1001/archinte.1991.00400110123024] [PMID: 1953234]

[116] Gordon, D.W.; Rosenthal, G.; Hart, J.; Sirota, R.; Baker, A.L. Chaparral Ingestion. *JAMA,* **1995**, *273*(6), 489-490.
[http://dx.doi.org/10.1001/jama.1995.03520300063038] [PMID: 7837368]

[117] Sheikh, N.M.; Philen, R.M.; Love, L.A. Chaparral-associated hepatotoxicity. *Arch. Intern. Med.,* **1997**, *157*(8), 913-919.
[http://dx.doi.org/10.1001/archinte.1997.00440290099011] [PMID: 9129552]

[118] Katz, M.; Saibil, F. Herbal hepatitis. *J. Clin. Gastroenterol.,* **1990**, *12*(2), 203-206.
[http://dx.doi.org/10.1097/00004836-199004000-00021] [PMID: 2324485]

[119] Kauma, H.; Koskela, R.; Mäkisalo, H.; Autio-Harmainen, H.; Lehtola, J.; Höckerstedt, K. Toxic acute hepatitis and hepatic fibrosis after consumption of chaparral tablets. *Scand. J. Gastroenterol.,* **2004**, *39*(11), 1168-1171.
[http://dx.doi.org/10.1080/00365520410007926] [PMID: 15545179]

[120] Stickel, F.; Patsenker, E.; Schuppan, D. Herbal hepatotoxicity. *J. Hepatol.,* **2005**, *43*(5), 901-910.
[http://dx.doi.org/10.1016/j.jhep.2005.08.002] [PMID: 16171893]

[121] Castot, A.; Larrey, D. Hepatitis observed during a treatment with a drug or tea containing wild germander. evaluation of 26 cases reported to the regional centers of pharmacovigilance. *Gastroenterol. Clin. Biol.,* **1992**, *16*(12), 916-922.
[PMID: 1493896]

[122] Larrey, D.; Vial, T.; Pauwels, A.; Castot, A.; Biour, M.; David, M.; Michel, H. Hepatitis after germander (*Teucrium chamaedrys*) administration: Another instance of herbal medicine hepatotoxicity. *Ann. Intern. Med.,* **1992**, *117*(2), 129-132.
[http://dx.doi.org/10.7326/0003-4819-117-2-129] [PMID: 1605427]

[123] Benninger, J.; Schneider, H.T.; Schuppan, D.; Kirchner, T.; Hahn, E.G. Acute hepatitis induced by greater celandine (*Chelidonium majus*). *Gastroenterology,* **1999**, *117*(5), 1234-1237.
[http://dx.doi.org/10.1016/S0016-5085(99)70410-5] [PMID: 10535888]

[124] Gori, L.; Galluzzi, P.; Mascherini, V.; Gallo, E.; Lapi, F.; Menniti-Ippolito, F.; Raschetti, R.; Mugelli, A.; Vannacci, A.; Firenzuoli, F. Two contemporary cases of hepatitis associated with *Teucrium chamaedrys L.* decoction use: Case reports and review of literature. *Basic Clin. Pharmacol. Toxicol.,* **2011**, *109*(6), 521-526.
       [http://dx.doi.org/10.1111/j.1742-7843.2011.00781.x] [PMID: 21848806]

CHAPTER 3

Bioactive Compounds from Plants Having Hepatoprotective Activity

Retno Widyowati[1,2,*], Rosita Handayani[1,2] and Ram Kumar Sahu[3]

[1] *Department of Pharmaceutical Science, Faculty of Pharmacy, Universitas Airlangga, Surabaya, 60115, Indonesia*

[2] *Natural Product Drug Discovery and Development Research Group, Faculty of Pharmacy, Universitas Airlangga, Surabaya, 60115, Indonesia*

[3] *Department of Pharmaceutical Sciences, Hemvati Nandan Bahuguna Garhwal University (A Central University), Chauras Campus, Tehri Garhwal-249161, Uttarakhand, India*

Abstract: The liver plays an essential role in metabolic management, and detoxification associating the metabolisms of toxins, lipids, alcohols, carbohydrates and various drugs. It also plays a role in the immune response. However, some conditions, such as viral infections (hepatitis), inflammation, continuous liquor consumption, periodic use of antibiotic-related drugs, and non-alcoholic fatty liver illness, can produce free radicals and cytokines, enhance lipid peroxidation, and induce damage to hepatocytes. Hepatoprotective agents are often the treatment of choice to improve liver function and protect the liver from exposure to harmful compounds. Based on scientific reports, *Silybum marianum*, *Moringa oleifera*, *Garcinia mangostana*, *Glycyrrhiza glabra*, *Mangifera indica*, *Amaranthus spinosus*, *Andrographis paniculata*, *Phyllanthus species* (*amarus, niruri, emblica*), *Curcuma species* (*longa, xanthorrhiza, manga*), and *Citrus species* (aurantium, sinensis, unshiu, grandis) have been broadly administered for the liver ailments therapy through antioxidant-associated abilities. Impressive studies have exposed that the health-promoting outcomes of bioactive constituents derived from plants have often been applied to their antioxidant characteristics and raise the cellular antioxidant protection system, scavenge free radicals, suppress lipid peroxidation, stimulate anti-inflammatory capacity, and assure the liver from destruction. These compounds are chlorogenic acid, curcumin, quercetin, hesperidin, rutin, betalains, apigenin, silymarin, phyllanthin, mangiferin, α-mangostin, bellidifolin, ginsenosides, glycyrrhizin, lycopene, and andrographolide.

Keywords: Clinical study, Flavonoids, Hepatoprotective, Human & health, *In vitro*, *In vivo*, Lignan, Phenolics, Saponin, Terpenoid, Xanthone.

---

* **Corresponding author Retno Widyowati:** Department of Pharmaceutical Science, Faculty of Pharmacy, Universitas Airlangga, Surabaya, 60115, Indonesia & Natural Product Drug Discovery and Development Research Group, Faculty of Pharmacy, Universitas Airlangga, Surabaya, 60115, Indonesia; Email: rr-retno-w@ff.unair.ac.id

INTRODUCTION

The liver is a central organ in the body's metabolism, and it is essential for survival in the form of protection, detoxification, and metabolism. It is the first organ after the digestive tract to be exposed to toxic materials, so it has the potential to be damaged and can lead to inflammation of liver cells and even cell death [1]. The prevalence of liver disease and its effects continue to increase. Liver disease is a world health problem, and more than 350 million people worldwide suffer from the disease [2]. Liver disease is commonly caused by infection and chemical compounds that enter the body through various mechanisms. One of the leading causes of the development of liver disease is an increase in stress which can be estimated as an imbalance between reactive oxygen species (ROS) production and antioxidant defense level [3].

The mechanism of liver disease begins with increased steatosis, and eventually, liver fibrosis can lead to death. Although the pathogenesis of fibrosis is unclear, ROS has a role in pathological changes in the liver, especially in liver disease problems caused by alcohol and toxins. Cell membranes have a significant role in countering the effects of ROS, the reaction process of peroxides into unsaturated fatty acids in the membrane can cause a decrease in membrane integrity and function, which implies quite severe pathological changes, as the natural protective mechanisms in the reduction of liver damage caused by peroxides. However, additional protective mechanisms through antioxidants are needed due to impaired protection or increasing oxygen species (OR). Many natural ingredients have antioxidant agents and are recommended to prevent and treat liver disease caused by free radicals [4].

Medicinal plants have been generally used to treat various types of liver diseases such as hepatitis, liver cirrhosis, jaundice, tumors or cancer, liver failure, cholangitis, leptospirosis, liver abscess, metabolic and degenerative lesions, and liver cell necrosis [5]. Medicinal plants have an essential contribution to human health that is promotive, therapeutic, and rehabilitative and it also contributes to disease prevention. The benefits of natural ingredients that have a role in traditional medicine have been generally developed. The use of natural or herbal ingredients has an essential role in treating cases of liver disease. Herbs can be assumed to have a hepatoprotective effect if they can maintain liver cell function and help accelerate healing. The use of herbs as hepatoprotective can be evaluated through antioxidant mechanisms. In Indonesia, some plants are believed to have efficacy as herbal plants. Therefore, Indonesia has an excellent opportunity to process medicinal plants into a product that provides hepatoprotection.

Hepatoprotector is a compound or substance that can protect cells and repair liver tissue disease by toxic effects. In its structure, hepatoprotective compounds include phenylpropanoids, coumarins, lignins, essential oils, terpenoids, saponins, flavonoids, lipid organic acids, alkaloids, and xanthines. Several natural antioxidant compounds such as flavonoids, terpenoids, and steroids have been studied pharmacologically for hepatoprotective activity [6]. This chapter hopes that scientific information can be obtained about herbal plants that have shown activity as hepatoprotection.

BIO MARKERS TO ASSESS THE LIVER DAMAGE AND HEPATOPROTECTIVE POTENCY

The Role of Antioxidant Enzymes in Liver Damage

Alcohol and some drugs can induce oxidative stress by increasing cellular oxidation, lipid peroxidation, and antioxidant depletion in the liver [7]. The body responds to chemical-induced damage by activating a set of endogenous antioxidant enzymes. Antioxidant enzymes provide protection by scavenging the ROS. Superoxide dismutase (SOD) catalyzes the conversion of superoxide radicals ($\cdot O_2$) to hydrogen peroxide (H_2O_2) [10]. Although H_2O_2 is not radical, it is rapidly converted by the Fenton reaction to the highly reactive $\cdot OH$ radical. Glutathione peroxidase (GPx) detoxifies H_2O_2 by reaction with glutathione (GSH) to produce oxidized glutathione (GSSG). The oxidized glutathione is then reduced to GSH by glutathione reductase (GSR). Catalase (CAT) neutralizes H_2O_2 into H_2O, reducing free radicals [11]. Heme oxygenase 1 (HO-1) is an isozyme that is required in phase II detoxification and has an important role during oxidative stress resistance.

In excessive oxidation conditions, the activity of this antioxidant enzyme will be affected. Decreased GSH, SOD, GPx, CAT, GSR, and HO-1 in hepatocytes causes cells to be more susceptible to the dangers posed by free radicals. This means that measuring antioxidant enzyme activity is an indirect method commonly used to assess the status of antioxidant defenses against ROS damage [11]. A compound that has the potential to be hepatoprotective will show an increase in the level/activity of this antioxidant enzyme, and most of them are antioxidants. Antioxidant compounds can protect the liver by scavenging ROS and neutralizing lipid peroxides (LPO). The main product of LPO processes is lipid hydroperoxides (LOOH), and the secondary product formed during LPO is malondialdehyde (MDA). Increasing secondary oxidation products (including MDA) upon lipid peroxidation in hepatic tissue will cause cellular damage and cell membrane disruption and deplete endogenous antioxidant enzymes [11].

The transcription factor-erythroid 2-related factor 2 (Nrf2) regulates the expression of antioxidant genes such as catalase, SOD, NADPH quinoneoxidoreductase 1, GPx, and heme oxygenase 1 (HO-1) [12, 13]. Up-regulation of antioxidant genes by Nrf2 t can inhibit free radicals' development and the expression of pro-inflammatory cytokines [14]. Therefore, Nrf2 can be used as a signaling target that controls oxidative stress and improves the inflammatory process [15].

Inflammation and Liver Damage

Some pathogens and chemical inducers can also trigger a systemic inflammatory response that triggers liver damage. This process occurs due to excessive oxidative stress, infiltration of immune cells in the liver, and prolonged release of inflammatory mediators. The entry of pathogens and chemicals induces liver damage and activates a variety of signaling pathways, including the activated nuclear factor kappa-light-chain-enhancer of activated B cells (NF-κB), mitogen-activated protein kinases (MAPKs), Janus kinases/signal transducers and transcriptional activators (JAKs)/STATS [15 - 17]. The accumulation of ROS causes oxidative stress in various cell organelles and promotes the development of inflammation. ROS can activate NF-κB, causing the up-regulation of various pro-inflammatory mediators and cytokines, such as interleukin-1 beta (IL-1β), tumor necrosis factor-alpha (TNF-α), and inducible nitric oxide synthase (iNOS), which play an essential role in the process of inflammation and cause liver tissue injury [18]. TNF-α is a potent pro-inflammatory cytokine that can trigger the production of other cytokines as well. In the liver, TNF-α, together with other cytokines, can attract inflammatory cells into the organ and destroy hepatocytes. Usually, the liver and other tissues can produce only small amounts of TNF-α. However, TNF-α experienced a significant increase in patients with liver disease [19]. The inflammatory process will cause further liver damage, so compounds with a hepatoprotective effect are expected to suppress the inflammatory response by down-regulating genes and mediators that play a role in this inflammatory process.

Apoptosis and Liver Damage

Liver cells can regenerate if damaged by ischemia, viral infection, alcohol, and reactive oxygen species (ROS). However, chronic exposure to hepatotoxic compounds can lead to increased cell death (apoptosis) that exacerbates the damage. In addition to fragments of DNA that reflect apoptosis, higher oxidative stress also resulted in increased cytochrome c production with subsequent activation of caspase-9 and caspase-3 [20]. Apoptosis is programmed cell death commonly used to remove damaged cells and protect cells from external hazards such as viruses and hepatotoxic compounds. In acute conditions, apoptosis plays an essential role as a protector, but if the apoptotic process occurs excessively over a long period, it will cause permanent fibrosis and necrosis. Hepatocyte apoptosis occurs through two pathways, the extrinsic pathway, and the intrinsic pathway. The extrinsic pathway is triggered by signal transmission from death receptors (DR) bound to inducing ligands such as FasL, TNF-α, and TNF-related apoptosis-inducing ligand (TRAIL) in membrane cells. This receptor-ligand binding activates Fas-associated protein with death domain [FADD]) and apoptosis-inducing molecules (caspase-8) form a death-induced signaling complex (DISC) and activate effector caspases (caspases-3, -6, and -7) to trigger cell death [21].

The intrinsic mechanism of cell death begins with chemical damage-inducing compounds that activate the ER stress pathway, increase lysosomal permeability, and activate JNK. This process will initiate pro-apoptotic proteins such as Bax, Bim, Bad, and Bid, overpowering the antiapoptotic proteins (Bcl-xL, Bcl-2). Activating pro-apoptotic proteins causes the mitochondrial membrane to become permeable, triggering the entry of ions and solutes into the matrix so that the matrix swells and ruptures and then releases pro-apoptotic proteins to trigger massive cell death [22]. Massive apoptosis indicates acute liver damage, while persistent apoptosis indicates chronic liver disease [22].

Other Liver Damage Markers

AST and ALT, two transaminase enzymes, seem to be the more often utilized liver damage markers. Increased permeability of membranes on the cells of the liver is caused by oxidative stress, which releases ALT and AST into the bloodstream, making them biochemical markers of liver disease. An enzyme that is membrane-bound, alkaline phosphatase (ALP), has the potential to modify membrane permeability and transport metabolic compounds. In addition to being an important diagnostic sign for liver necrosis, lactate dehydrogenase (LDH) is an intracellular enzyme that increases in serum. In the antioxidant defense system, Gamma-glutamyltranspeptidase (GGT), positioned on the plasma membrane's outermost layer, serves a crucial role, and its serum concentration is a good indicator of oxidative stress and cellular damage. Damage to the hepatic tissue causes these enzymes to be released into the bloodstream, resulting in higher serum levels [23]. Increased blood-stream levels of ALT, ALAT, AST, aspartate aminotransferase (ASAT), ALP, and LDH are indications of severe hepatic cell necrosis [24]. The increased levels of ALT, AST, and γ-GT, as well as total and direct bilirubin, reflect cellular permeability and degradation of the liver cell membrane's functional integrity [25] and mitochondrial disturbance, respectively. An increase in transaminases along with an increase in bilirubin levels to more than double can be used as a reference to indicate the occurrence of liver damage [26]. The list of biomarkers that are commonly used to assess liver damage is resumed in Table **1**.

Table 1. Biomarkers to assess the liver damage.

Marker	Hepatoprotective action
Liver injury biomarkers (ALT, AST, ASAT, GGT, ALP, LDH)	Decrease (↓)
An antioxidant enzyme (SOD, GSH, GPx, CAT, γ-GT)	Increase (↑)
Oxidative stress marker (LOOH, LPO, TBARS/MDA, H2O2, 4-HNE)	Decrease (↓)
Extracellular regulated kinase (ERK), p38 MAPKs, c-Jun N-terminal kinase (JNK) inhibitor SP600125, and NQO1	
STAT3, TAK1, NF-κB	Inhibits/down-regulate (↓)
Inflammatory mediators, cytokines, chemokines (iNOS, TNF-α, interferon-γ, IL-1β/2/6)	Decrease (↓)
Antioxidant regulation (Nrf2)	Activate/up-regulate (↑)
Inflammatory signaling pathway (TLR4)	Inhibits/down-regulate (↓)
Pro-apoptotic proteins (Bax, Bim, Bad, Bid)	Decrease (↓)
Apoptotic indicator (DNA fragmentation)	Decrease (↓)
Apoptotic mediators (caspase-9 and caspase-3)	Decrease (↓)

Other important biomarkers such as α-fetoprotein, ferritin, and abnormal prothrombin were liver damage markers. Alpha-fetoprotein (AFP) or fetal protein is derived from the yolk sac and liver of the developing fetus and has the same molecular weight as albumin and 1-globulin. In 1963, serum AFP was used as a tumor marker for hepatocellular carcinoma (HCC) because its levels were elevated in patients with chronic liver disease (viral hepatitis) and non-hepatic malignancies (gastric, pancreatic, biliary, and germ cell tumors). AFP values >400 ng/ml indicate that the patient has HCC and he/she is at the fibrotic stage of chronic hepatitis C virus infection.

Ferritin is a protein with 24 heavy chains (H-ferritin) and light chain (FTL) subunits that function as the main iron storage protein, playing a role in proliferation, angiogenesis, and immunosuppression. Important FTLs for HCC immunity and TAA candidates were identified by recombinant cDNA expression library (SEREX) serological analysis. Serum ferritin (SF) levels are elevated in patients with nonalcoholic fatty liver disease (NAFLD) due to systemic inflammation, increased iron stores, or both. In severe NAFLD, patients had an SF value $> 1.5 \times$ ULN with steatosis, fibrosis, hepatocellular ballooning, and a diagnosis of NASH ($P < 0.026$).

Abnormal prothrombin in patients with acute liver failure (AHF) at higher levels than acute hepatitis can be determined by the latex-in-plasma agglutination method. Under these conditions, abnormal prothrombin concentrations are significantly higher than in acute liver failure because abnormal prothrombin concentrations are inversely related to hepaplastin tests or prothrombin time. Measurement of abnormal plasma prothrombin is useful for monitoring the severity of acute liver injury. Cross-immune electrophoresis can also detect abnormal prothrombin in ARF and disseminated intravascular coagulation syndrome which exhibits different mobility with PIVKA-II. This suggests that abnormal prothrombin may be a valuable marker for AHF.

HEPATOPROTECTIVE COMPOUNDS FROM NATURAL PRODUCTS

Hepatoprotective are compounds or substances that can protect cells and repair damaged liver tissues. There are phenolics, flavonoids, lignans, xanthines, saponins, and terpenoids.

Phenolics and Flavonoids

A comprehensive review of phenolics' role in hepatoprotection mechanism has been discussed [27]. Flavonoids, which act as antioxidants, free radical scavenging, and anti-lipoperoxidation agents, are helpful in hepatoprotection [28]. The hepatoprotective activity of some flavonoids has been studied. Chlorogenic acid, quercetin, hesperidin, betalain, and apigenin showed hepatoprotective activity whether in vitro or *in vivo*.

Chlorogenic Acid

Chlorogenic acid abbreviated as CGA comes from the hydroxycinnamic acid family in the form of polyphenol compounds that have a large number of hydroxyl groups (Fig. 1). CGA consists of a series of cinnamic hydroxyl esters together with quinic acid, covering caffeoyl-, coumaroyl quinic acid, feruloyl-, and dicaffeoyl-.

CGA protects against various metabolic disorders [29], some of which can relieve hepatic ischemia and reperfusion injury [30] through the inhibition of the LPS-induced pro-inflammatory response in low doses of injury and hepatic stellate cells [31]. CGA effectively suppresses LPS-induced pro-inflammatory reactions in HSCs that due to the LPS/ROS/NF-kB signaling pathway inhibition [31]. CGA reduces the energy stock of hepatic lipid metabolism, especially provided by glycolysis. Increased production of ATP energy will raise liver tissue protein synthesis, repair tissue destruction, and relieve oxidative stress. Thus, CGA can manage the metabolism of nutrients and gut microbiota conservation in unified multi-metabolic pathways [32]. So CGA inhibits α-glucosidase activity, improves cellular mechanisms, activates AMPK, ameliorates skeletal muscle GLUT4 expression, up-regulates hepatic PPAR-α, inhibits G-6-Pase expression and alters GIP concentrations [33].

CGA as caffeoylquinic acid is broadly contained in plants alike honeysuckle and apples as well as beverages such as coffee and tea [34, 35] and also other plants in the Asteraceae and Lamiaceae families. CGA has various isomeric forms. Different types of coffee extract contain different CGA isomers although the most widely amount of isomers present is about 10 g/100 g. Tajik *et al.* (2017) reported that green coffee beans contain 76-84% CGA. Then, other plants and natural products contain 3-CQA, 4-CQA (cryptochlorogenic acid), and 5-CQA (neochlorogenic acid) [36]. CGA is the main phenolic acid in *Moringa oleifera* leaves and is available in the form of esters of hydroxycinnamic acid (caffeic acid) and quinic acid [37]. It inhibits liver cell damage and reduces enzyme leakage into the blood so this plant extract is also able to reduce toxicity [38]. CGA is also contained in sunflower seeds (29.9-45.5 g/kg Dw), eggplants (14.1-28.0 g/kg Dw), mate tea (4.8-24.9 g/kg Dw), artichoke (1.1-1.8 g/kg Dw), pepper (0.7-0.9 g/kg Dw), plum (0.4 g/kg Dw), and tomato (0.2-0.4 g/kg Dw) [39].

Curcumin

Curcumin (Fig. **1**) is found in many *Curcuma species*. Many studies about the hepatoprotective effect of curcumin have been conducted. Pre- and post-treatment with 20 mg/kg of curcumin yielded a significant decrease in plasma malondialdehyde (MDA) and serum ALT. At the same time, SOD activity is being increased [40]. Administration of curcumin at a dose of 200 mg/kg for 3 days displayed significant liver damage protection by developing glutathione peroxidase and hepatic superoxide dismutase activity in rats induced by CCl_4 [41]. At a dose of 100 mg/kg for 5 days continuously by I.P. after methotrexate (MTX) treatment, curcumin could mitigate MTX injurious influences and repair all the changed biochemical parameters [42]. Curcumin at a dose of 80 mg/kg in rats induced by $CuSO_4$ displayed antioxidant enzymes (CAT, SOD, and GSH) improved by MDA decreasing in the liver [43].Curcumin as hepatoprotective has several mechanisms such as (1) Pp-regulation of the expression of Nrf2, SOD, CAT, and GSH; (2) Preventing the cytotoxic effect of NO as oxygen free radicals; and (3) Reducing inflammatory mediators and cytokines [44].

One of the plants that contain curcumin is *Curcuma longa*. The aqueous extract of this plant has hepatoprotective activity against carbon tetrachloride toxicity. Meanwhile, their ethanol extract can maintain or decrease the development of thioacetamide (TAA)-induced liver cirrhosis. The *Curcuma longa* extract as a hepatoprotective agent has mechanism for maintaining harmful cascade events caused by TAA toxicity. They also maintain the condition of the liver in terms of its function, structure, and properties towards venous. The curcumin in the extract is responsible for the hepatoprotective effect [45]. Other plants that contain curcumin are *Curcuma xanthorrhiza* and *Curcuma manga*.

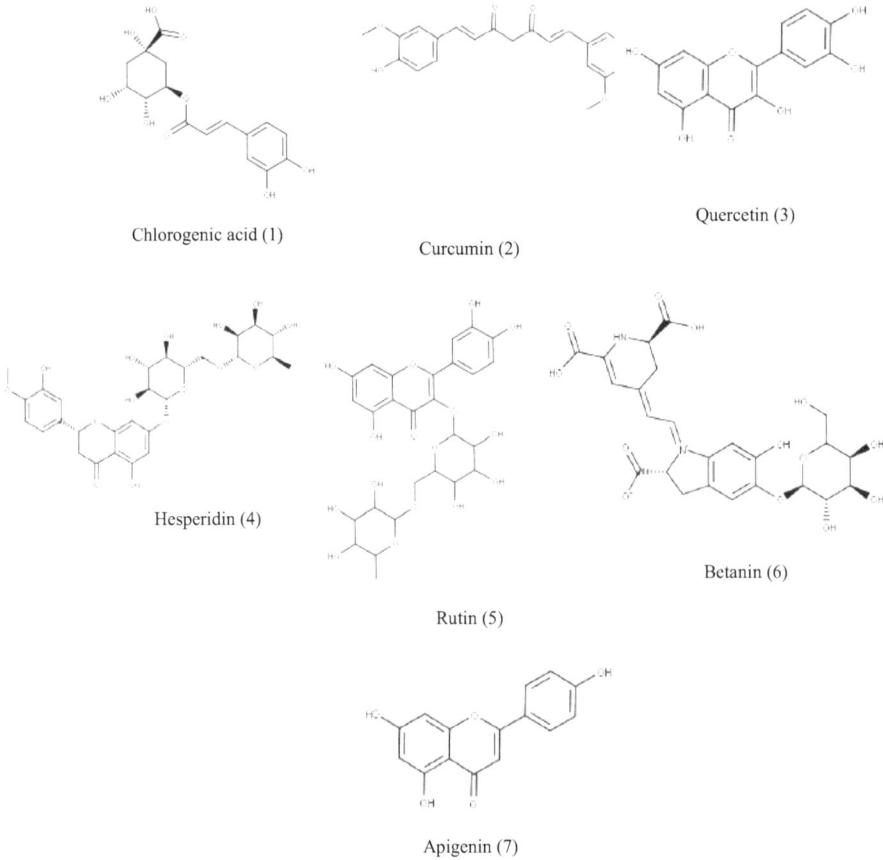

Chlorogenic acid (1)

Curcumin (2)

Quercetin (3)

Hesperidin (4)

Rutin (5)

Betanin (6)

Apigenin (7)

Fig. (1). Phenol and flavonoid compounds with hepatoprotective activity

Quercetin

Quercetin (Fig. **1**) is a common flavonoid in plants that shows its activities as an anti-inflammatory, anticancer, and antioxidant agent. Several studies use cellular, and animal models, and humans modulate pathways of signaling and gene expressions. The 50 mg/kg/day quercetin administered to male Wistar rats induced by carbon tetrachloride (CCl_4), decreased AST, ALT, conjugated bilirubin, total bilirubin levels in serum, and lipid peroxidation levels, and also increased the levels of SOD, catalase, GSH, GST, and GPx [46]. Co-treatment of Lindane and quercetin (10 mg/kg) significantly declined histology modification, renal and serum hepatic markers, and MDA. It also increased the condition of cellular antioxidants, repaired Lindane-induced oxidative stress in female albino Wistar rats' liver [47], and also repaired liver damage and histopathological changes. Quercetin restrains inflammatory cytokines release and is involved in Bax, Bcl-2, Beclin-1, LC3, P62, and caspase 9 expressions and also decreased TRAF6 and p-JNK expression. In the TRAF6/JNK pathway, quercetin constricted autophagy and apoptosis in ConA-induced autoimmune hepatitis [48].

Quercetin is commonly found in capers (233 mg/100g), mango (46.9 mg/100g), onions (22 mg/100g), cranberries (14 mg/100g), asparagus (7.61 mg/100g), apples (4.7 mg/100g), broccoli (2.51 mg/100g), green tea (2.69 mg/100g), and red grapes (1.38 mg/100g).

Hesperidin

Hesperidin (Fig. **1**) is a pharmacologically active flavonoid glucoside and is contained in citrus species such as orange, lime, lemon, and blood orange. Hesperidin in herbal formulations did not cause side effects and/or toxicity because its LD_{50} against orally acute toxicity test was higher than 2000 mg/kg [49].

Hesperidin at a dose of 200 mg/kg administered orally for one week in Male Wistar rats induced by CCl_4 showed significant hepatoprotective activity in decreasing ALT, AST, and TBARS (MDA), but increasing GSH, SOD, and CAT levels [50]. Another study using the same animal models with different chemical damage inducers (LPS, lipopolysaccharide) also showed the hepatoprotective of hesperidin at the same dose (200 mg/kg), marked by the decrease of AST, ALT, bilirubin, TBARS (MDA), and nitrite serum level. In contrast, the level of SOD and GPH has increased and the inhibition of cytokine by HDN is rare [51]. Hesperidin hepatoprotective mechanisms include increasing enzymatic and non-enzymatic antioxidant capacity, associated with anti-apoptotic and inflammatory factors. In addition to the mechanism, it can occur by lowering oxidative stress markers, liver enzymes, inflammatory factors, and apoptotic factors such as Bax,

Bad, and caspase 3 [49]. This compound also known as hesperetin--rhamnoglucoside is contained in many citrus species such as *Citrus unshiu*, *Citrus aurantium*L., and *Citrus sinensis* (Rutaceae). It is used for liver disease, and jaundice and to ameliorate sodium arsenite-induced toxicity in rats [52].

Rutin

Rutin (Fig. **1**) is a common flavonoid in the Rutaceae. In a study using Sprague-Dawley rats induced by CCl_4, 50 and 70 mg/kg of rutin significantly depleted the level of AST, γ-GT, ALP, and ALT in serum and also lipid peroxidation (TBARS/MDA), and increased endogenous liver antioxidant enzymes levels such as CAT, GPx, glutathione (GSH), SOD, glutathione reductase (GSR), and glutathione-S-transferase (GST). Rutin not only reduced DNA fragmentation and oxo8dG damage but also increased the expression of p53 and CYP2E1 in rats induced by CCl_4 [53].

Many fruits and peels, especially citrus fruits like *Ruta graveolens*, *Morus alba,* or *Citrus grandis*, contain rutin, which is generated by higher plants. Buckwheat and Asparagus are examples of medicinal plants that are rich in rutin, commonly known as vitamin P. In addition, Buckwheat (*Fagopyrum esculentum*) is one of the best common sources of food [54]. This compound is also found in *Rhus cotinus* (10.53%), green tea (10.18%), grape (10.16%), betulae pendula leaves (5.54%), geranium (2.28%), arpnia (0.34%), cherry (0.18%), apple (0.17%), and red pepper (0.17%) [55].

Betalains

Betalains are pigments contained in *Beta vulgaris* var. Rubra, known as red beetroot, and in several other plant species, for example, Amaranthus. The most abundant betalain component around 75-95% is betanin or betanidin 5-O-β--glucoside (Fig. **1**) [56]. Red beetroot extract is reported to prevent liver damage that is chlorpyrifos (CPF)-induced and inhibits inflammation, oxidative stress, and apoptosis. The administration of 300 mg/kg of red beetroot extract for 28 days prevented CPFinduced liver damage through the recreation of inflammation, apoptosis, and oxidative stress. This is accompanied by decreasing AST, ALP, ALT, bilirubin, LPO, iNOS, NO, and pro-inflammatory cytokine serum levels. Red beetroot extract also prevented changes in CPF-induced histological and boosted GSH, antioxidant enzymes, Bcl-2, and Nrf2 expression, whereas caspase-3 and Bax were decreased [57]. Han *et al.* [58] showed that betanin at doses of 25 and 100 mg/kg could reduce AST, MDA, and ALT serum levels and increase SOD, CAT, and GSH activities in the male Sprague-Dawley rats induced by paraquat. The hepatoprotective activity mechanism may appear as CYP 3A2 expression and mitochondria protection [58].

Betalains are basic ingredients of natural food coloring used in the manufacture of modern food and are water-soluble pigments. These compounds give color to flowers and fruits and consist of yellow betaxanthins and red-purple betacyanins that mainly originated from Caryophyllales plants. *Amaranthus spinosus* is rich in betalains exhibiting antidiabetic effects by reducing glycemia up to 40% without inducing liver damage and weight loss. Currently, these dyes can be encouraged as synthetic dye alternatives for food additives. The list of plants that produce betalain is presented in Table **2**.

Table 2. Betalain produced from several plants [59].

Family	Species	Betalains
Amaranthaceae	*Amaranthus spinosus*	Amaranthine & isoamaranthine
	Gomphrena globosa	Betaxanthins& several betacyanins
	Celosia argentea (var.plumoseand var.cristata)	Amaranthine, betalamic acid, dopamine-derived betacyanins
Cactaceae	*Hylocereus polyrhizus*	Betacyanins, bougainvillean-r-l, betanin, isobetanin, isophyllocactin, phyllocactin, &hylocerenin
Aizoaceae	*Lampranthus productus*	Dopaxanthin, betanidin

Supplements containing raw red beet juice reduce LDL-c, total cholesterol, and non-HDL-c. In addition, betanin was treated in AML mice indicating reduced LDL levels and short-chain fatty acid (SCFA) production. Chips containing 3% RBR inhibited the growth of TC and TAG also reduced liver TC levels, thereby affecting metabolism dyslipidemia.

Apigenin

Apigenin (4', 5, 7,-trihydroxyflavone in Fig. (**7**) is contained in *Hypericum perforatum* buds and flowers, oranges, parsley, onions, tea, chamomile, sprouts, and wheat. Chamomile made from *Matricaria chamomilla* dried flowers is one of the most common apigenins consumed as herbal tea with a single ingredient. A chamomile infusion usually contains 0.8-1.2% of apigenin and essential oils with the characteristic flavoring, aromatic, and coloring properties. Another source for apigenin is red wine grapes.

In vivo, apigenin significantly reduces AST and ALT activity in mice serum CCl_4-induced, lipid peroxidation, and MDA in liver tissue. Increased GSH and GPx, as well as increased SOD and CAT levels, indicate these actions. Apigenin also improved inflammation through IL-6 and TNF-α downregulation and IL-10 upregulation. Employing Western blot, real-time qPCR, and immunofluorescence assays, apigenin boosted cellular inhibitor of apoptosis protein (c-IAP) 1 and TNF receptor-associated factor (TRAF) 2/3, improved NF-B-inducing kinase (NIK), and promoted nuclear translocation of NF-B2 [60]. Apigenin reduces oxidative stress that is inflammation-induced in tissues by regulating blood enzyme markers, interleukins, various oxidative stress markers, and several other related enzyme expressions. Apigenin's antioxidant effect is regulated by an increase in the supply of antioxidant enzymes in the body [61].

Lignans

Lignans have 2,3-dibenzylbutane structures that include a phenolic dimer. As minor constituents in plants, lignans form the building blocks for lignin formation in plant cell walls. Some lignans that have hepatoprotective activity are silymarin and phyllanthin.

Sylimarin

Silymarin is a compound extracted from milk thistle plant seeds such as *Silybum marianum* L and this plant also contains seven flavonolignans and taxifolin (flavonoid) [62]. This compound works by regulating enzymes related to hepatocyte cellular damage and is a free radical scavenger. It also has hepatoprotective effects as shown in clinical studies for non-alcoholic or alcoholic fatty liver disease patients, along with cirrhosis patients. Silymarin also inhibited interferon-γ, IL-2, and TNF-α production via increased T cells isolated and peripheral blood mononuclear cells from infected and non-infected hepatitis C virus [63]. Some studies showed ALT development and others showed no effect. Then one study indicated no improvement of histological effect without a biochemical response. There is no information about low to high doses of silymarin for hepatoprotection [62]. The mechanism of silymarin/silybin against Non-alcoholic fatty liver disease (NAFLD) development by involved several therapeutic targets [64].

There are eight main components obtained from silymarin, namely taxifolin (2%), isosilychristin (2%), isosilybin B (4%), isosilybin A (6%), silychristin (12%), silybin A (16%), silydianin (16%), and silybin B (24%) (Fig. **2**). A plant containing silymarin lower than 100% means that the extract contains silymarin between 70% and 80%, and the remainder contains polyphenols and aliphatic fatty acids (palmitic and oleic acids).

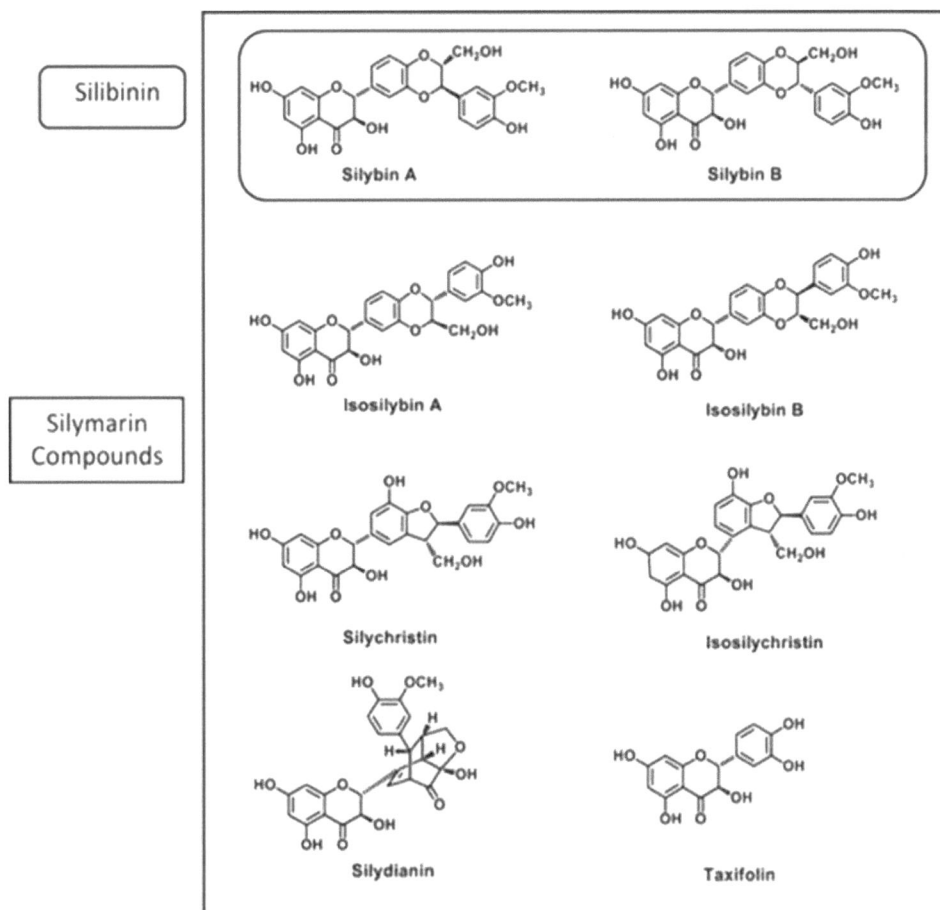

Fig. (2). Several kinds of silymarin compounds

Phyllanthin

Phyllanthin (Fig. **3**) is widely distributed in Phyllanthus species. Various studies have confirmed its hepatoprotective potency in pre-clinical tests [65 - 68]. A specific study showed that phyllanthinprevents the diethylnitrosamine (DEN) effect in mice by repairing all oxidative DNA damage, liver function enzymes, and tumor-specific markers by leading to caspase-dependent apoptosis via the signaling pathway of mTOR/PI3K and increased anti-oxidant capacity [67].

Phyllanthus niruri has the potential to be hepatoprotective. Treatment with this plant significantly reduces the toxic effects of TAA as follows: 1) Eliminates TAA-causing stimuli, neutralizes ROS using a high dose, and depresses endogenous enzymes until normal levels; 2) Keeps the HSC at rest; and 3)

Increased TIMP1 release to counterbalance MMP2 then accomplished hepatocyte cellular system remodeling that maintains shape liver function and appearance in normal conditions. *Phyllanthus niruri* protects liver function by activating HSCs by increasing EMC such as Colla, TGFb, MMP2, and TIMP1 [69].

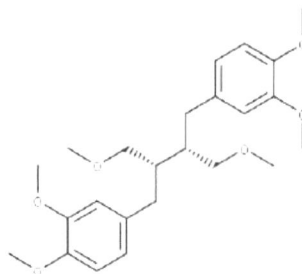

Fig. (3). Structure of phyllanthin

Xanthones

Xanthen-9H-ones (dibenzo-gamma-pirone) are secondary metabolites that include the xanthones group and are commonly discovered in plants, lichens, and fungi. The structure and chromatographic profile of xanthones are similar to those of flavonoids but are found in limited quantities in nature and consist of oxygenated heterocycles whose role is in medicinalchemistry. Xanthones are found in the families Gentianaceae, Guttiferae, Moraceae, Clusiaceae, and Polygalaceae. One example of a plant containing xanthonesfrom the Guttiferae family is *Garcinia mangostana*. Mangiferin, α-mangostin, 1,7-dihydroxy-3,4,8-trimethoxyxanthone, and bellidifolin are part of the xanthones that have hepatoprotective activity.

Mangiferin

The 2-C-β-D-glucopyranosyl-1,3,6,7-tetrahydroxyxanthone or mangiferin (Fig. **4**) as xanthone is generally found in *Mangifera indica* bark and leaves. Administration of 25 mg/Kg mangiferin to acetaminophen-induced mice could potentially reduce the lipid peroxidation, ALT, AST, and increase the SOD and GSH stages. The p-JNK and AMPK down-regulation was also observed, increasing p47 phox mRNA expression and HO-1 protein. Mangiferin also suppresses the inflammatory genes such as IL-6, TNF-α, MCP-1, CXCL-2, and CXCL-1 in basal stages. Mangiferin has mechanism for hepatoprotective actions by developing acetaminophen and APAP-Cys adduct formation metabolism complied by inflammation and JNK-mediated oxidative stress [70]. Another study using mangiferin at different doses also showed similar effects. It is observed that mangiferin could decrease serum GPx activity and liver and serum lipid peroxidation, and also increase serum SOD, serum and liver GSH [71, 72].

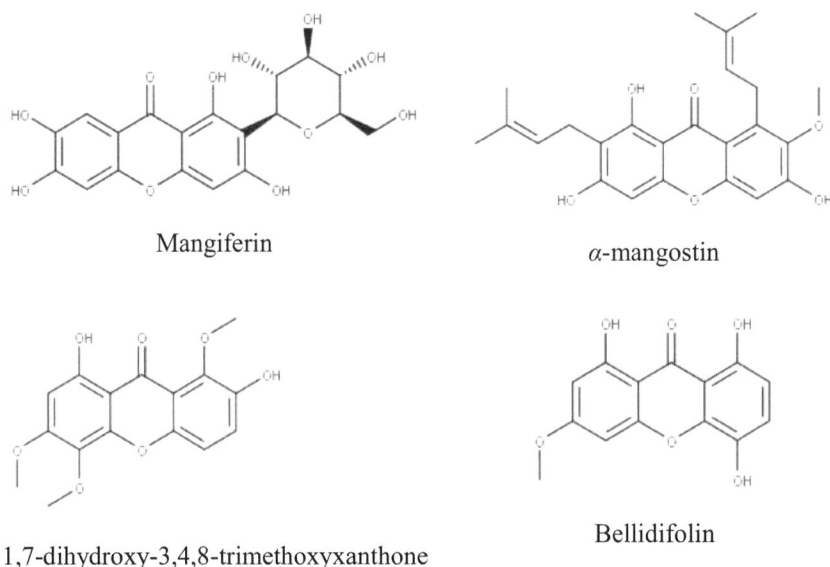

Fig. (4). Xanthone compounds with hepatoprotective activity

α-mangostin

The α-mangostin (Fig. **4**) is a natural xanthones from *Garcinia mangostana* L [73]. A study showed that the administration of α-mangostin with a dose of 12.5 and 25 mg/kg daily for 6 days in acetaminophen-induced could decrease ALT, AST, IL-1β, TNF-α, IL-6, and MDA serum levels; and recovered GSH, SOD, CAT activities. The pretreatment of α-mangostin also hindered infiltration of inflammatory cells, acetaminophen-induced hepatocellular necrosis, and hyperemia. Furthermore, ERK, IL-1β, JNK, p38 MAPK, IL-6, and TNF-α expression are being depleted [74].

1,7-dihydroxy-3,4,8-trimethoxyxanthone and Bellidifolin

Bellidifolin and 1,7-dihydroxy-3,4,8 trimethoxyxanthone (Fig. **4**) were extracted from the stems of *Swertia punicea*. They showed significant hepatoprotective activity against carbon tétrachlorides-induced HepG2 cell damage, and significantly reduced AST, LDH and MDA. Dimethylnitrosamine (DMN)-induced fibrotic rats received 1,7-dihydroxy-3,4,8-trimethoxyxanthone orally, which reversed the rise of ALT, AST, and total bilirubin [75].

Saponins

Saponins are included in the steroid and triterpenoid glycosides found in many plant species. Derived from the Latin *sapo* that means soap, because it has surfactant properties to form foam. Several saponins that have hepatoprotection activity areginsenosides and glycyrrhizin.

Ginsenosides

Ginsenosides (Fig. **5**) are the essential active constituents contained in *Panax ginseng* Meyer. A study showed the hepatoprotective activity of ginsenoside Rg1 in induced-Dgalactose (D-gal) mice. At a dose of 10 mg/kg ginsenoside Rg1 significantly suppressed ALT, MDA, and AST elevation and also significantly escalated the oxidative enzymes such as GSH-Px and SOD. Furthermore, hepatocyte degenerative alterations and liver damage were decreased. Ginsenoside Rg1 also gives D-gal-induced liver damage protection in mice via decreasing DNA damage, reducing the AGE content, blocking oxidative stress, and decreasing DNA damage [76]. Another study showed that administration of ginsenoside Rg1 at doses of 15, 30, and 60 mg/kg in mice induced by CCl_4 could decrease the inflammation response of the liver *via* suppressing inflammation-related genes expression levels, including IL-1β, TNF-α, IL-6, iNOS, and COX-2. Furthermore, ginsenoside Rg1 increased liver detoxification abilities by up-regulating Nrf2 and anti-oxidative stress [77]. When ginseng is heated, it will produce ginsenoside Rk1. The administration of ginsenoside Rk1 in paracetamol induced-mice at a dose of 10 mg/kg or 20 mg/kg for 7 days could suppress apoptotic pathways by reducing Bax protein expression levels and stimulating Bcl-2. It also reversed inflammatory infiltration in liver tissues and paracetamol-induced necrosis [78]. Although many studies confirm its hepatoprotective activity, some ginseng components showed CYP3A4 inhibition. Consequently, when Ginseng extract or ginsenosides are applied clinically with other drugs, it should be scrutinized to define the inhibition of a particular CYP450 enzyme that is responsible fordrug metabolism. It might lead to stimulated efficacy and finally severe hepatotoxicity [79].

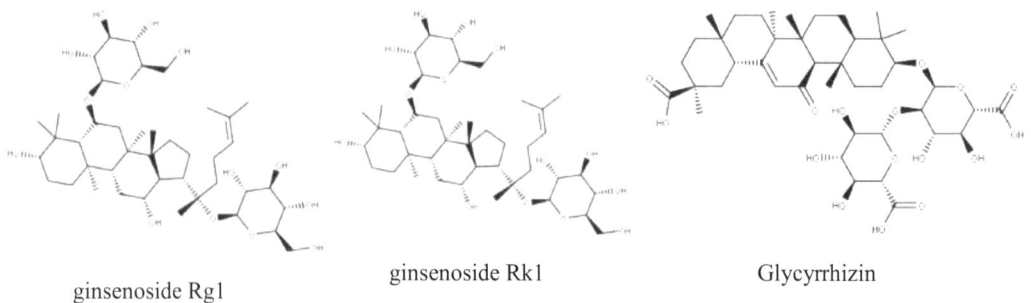

ginsenoside Rg1   ginsenoside Rk1   Glycyrrhizin

Fig. (5). Saponin compounds with hepatoprotective activity

Glycyrrhizin

Glycyrrhizin (Fig. **5**) also called Glycyrrhizic acid is triterpene glycoside (saponins) and is commonly found in *Glycyrrhiza glabra* (licorice) root. It has been improved as a hepatoprotective drug in Japan and China and producesthe same pharmacological effects [80]. Since 1979, Japan has glycyrrhizin injections for chronic hepatitis [81]. It significantly reduces hepatocellular carcinoma incidence of IFN-resistant active chronic hepatitis C patients whose value of average aminotransferase was twice or more of normal condition after interferon. *In vivo* experiments, glycyrrhizin reduces the inflammatory cytokines production of IL-1, IL-6, and TNF-α [82].

Terpenoids

Terpenoids are natural hydrocarbon compounds and polymer derivatives of isoprene units (C_5H_8). This compound is found in all essential oils and combined resins of plant or animal origin. Several plants provide protection from liver damage caused by toxic chemicals, drug screening models, and their oxidative mechanisms. The liver-protective activity of the plant has a mechanism of action related to its antioxidant potential and hepatoprotective safety. Terpenoids become one of the important compounds that act as antioxidants, and allopathic agents in hepatoprotection, one of which is andrographolide.It is very effective in the treatment of hepatitis, jaundice, and liver failure.

Lycopene

Lycopene (Fig. **6**) is a lipophilic red-colored terpene commonly found in *Solanum lycopersicum*. The hepatoprotective effect of 5, 10, and 20 mg/kg of lycopene has been studied in High Fat Diet-induced male Wistar rats, and the level of AST, ALT, and MDA significantly decreased, whereas SOD and GSH significantly increased in a dose-dependent manner. Then, the TNF-α expression and CYP2E1 also reduce [83].

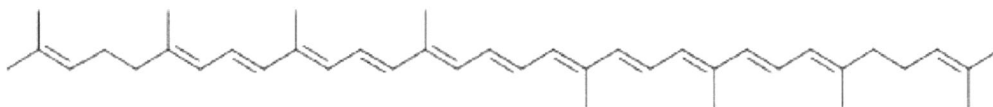

Fig. (6). Structure of lycopene

Andrographolide

Andrographolide (Fig. **7**) is an extremely bitter diterpenoid, first isolated from *Andrographis paniculata* [84]. A study of andrographolide in carbon tetrachloride

(CCl$_4$)-induced rats resulted in that andrographolide could prevent liver injury by inhibiting the inflammatory responses and oxidative stress. The hepatoprotective effect of andrographolide is particularly marked by a significant decrease in AST levels, serum ALT, TNF-α, and hepatic MDA activity, along with a remarkable increase in heme oxygenase-1 (HO-1) transcriptional and hepatic GSH content [85].

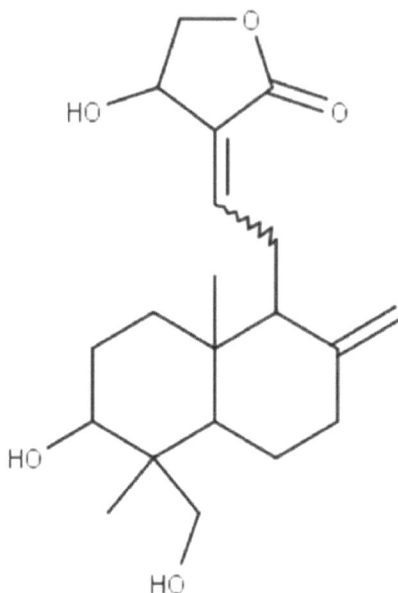

Fig. (7). Structure of andrographolide

HEPATOPROTECTIVE ASSAY

In vitro Activity Assay

Hepatocytes are isolated in situ under aseptic conditions and deposited in chilled HEPES (N-2-hydroxyethylpiperazine-N-2-ethanesulphonic acid). Then, hepato-cytes were isolated and expose to test samples and chemical inducer liver damage such as paracetamol, CCl$_4$, ethanol, *etc.* In the specified time period, the toxicity or protection degree is assessed through enzyme levels (ALT, AST, SOD, GSH, GPx), viability test, and protein expression [86]. An overview of the in vitro hepatoprotective test method is shown in Fig. (**8**) and the plants that have the potential to be hepatoprotective are summarized in Table **3**.

Table 3. *In vitro* **hepatoprotective activity studies of natural product.**

Name (plant)	Bioactive compound	Part used	In vitro model, liver damage inducer	Tested concentration	Hepatoprotective effects	Ref
Cleome viscosa L.	visconoside C (flavonol glycoside)	Leaf	HepG2 cells, CCl$_4$	100 μM	↑ cell viability in CCl4 induced cells (note: At 25 μM and 50 μM showed cytotoxic activity against HepG2 cells)	[88]
Panax ginseng Mayer	ginsenoside-Rg2 (G-Rg2) and -Rh1 (G-Rh1)		HepG2 cells, LPS	25-100 μg/ml, LPS	↓STAT3, ↓TAK1, ↓JNK, ↓ NF-Kb	[15]
Ziziphus jujube Mill	Maslinic Acid		Liver Slice Culture, CCl$_4$	100 g/mL extract 10 g/mL Maslinic Acid	↓LDH units, ↓SOD units, ↓CAT units, ↓ LPO	[11]
Citrus grandis	Coumarin compounds: columbianoside, meranzin hydrate I.	Pericarp	LO2 cells, D-galactosamine.	20 μM	↓ALT, ↓AST, ↓MDA, ↑SOD, ↑GSH-Px	[89]
Murraya koenigii	Alkaloids: (1′R,3′R,4′R,6′S)-endocycliomurrayamine-A, claulansiums A, 1′-Omethylclaulamine B, Dunnine E	Whole plants	HL-7702 cells, D-galactosamine	10 μM	↑cell survival rate	[90]
Hancornia speciosa	Rutin, chlorogenic acid	Fruit	L929 cell line, H$_2$O$_2$	10 50 g/mL	↓LPO, ↓MDA	[91]
Terminalia chebula	chebulinic acid	Fruit	L-02 cell line, t-BHP	26 μM	↓ROS, ↑HO-1, ↑NQO1, ↑Nrf2, ↑ERK, ↑JNK, ↑MAPKs	[92]
Terminalia chebula	chebulinic acid	Fruit	Transgenic zebrafish larvae, acetaminophen	26 μM	protected zebrafish larvae from acetaminophen toxicity	[92]

(Table 3) cont.....

Name (plant)	Bioactive compound	Part used	In vitro model, liver damage inducer	Tested concentration	Hepatoprotective effects	Ref
Crocus sativus	*Kaempferol glucosides	Petals	normal rat liver cell line (BRL-3A), t-BHP	25, 50, and 100 µg/mL	↑cell survival rate, ↓ROS, ↓ALT, ↓AST, ↓LDH, ↑SOD, ↑GSH, ↑CAT. ↑SOD, ↑HO-1, ↑Keap-1, ↑Nrf2, ↓INOS, ↓IL-6, ↓NF-Kb, ↓caspase-3, ↓caspase-9	[93]
Garcinia mangostana L	γ-mangostin	Peel	HL-7702 cells, t-BHP	0.63-5.00 µM	↓ALT, ↓AST, ↓MDA, ↓LPO,↓ROS, ↑SOD, ↑GSH,	[94]
Phyllanthus amarus Schum	phyllanthin	Not mentioned	Primary culture of rat hepatocytes, ethanol	1-4 4 µg/ml	↓ALT, ↓AST, ↓ROS, ↓MDA, ↑SOD, ↑GSH, ↑GPx, ↑CAT, ↑GR, ↑GST	[65]
Phyllanthus sp.	phyllanthin	Not mentioned	HepG2, Doxorubicin	1-30 µM	↑apoptosis, No toxicity observed in the normal HL7702 cells	[69, 95]
Ganoderma lucidum	*triterpenoids	Fruiting bodies	HepG2 cells, t-BHP	200 µg/ml	↓ALT, ↓AST, ↓LDH, ↓MDA, ↑SOD, ↑GSH	[96]

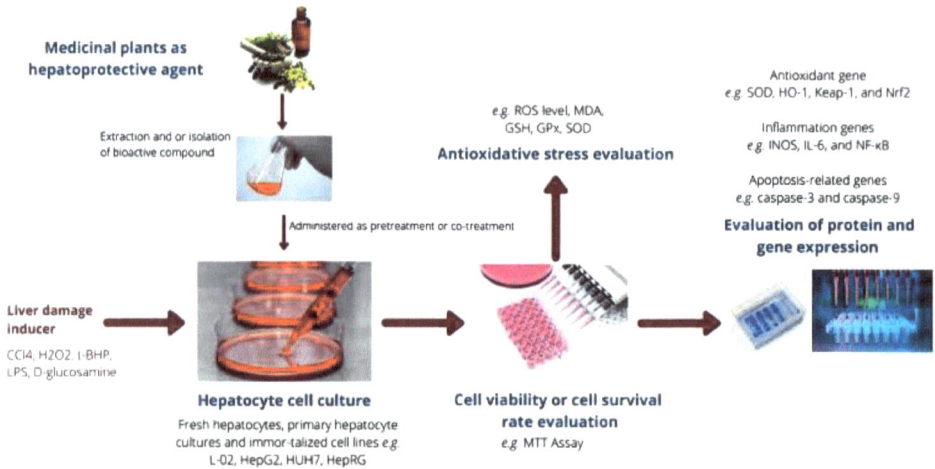

Fig. (8). Common method of *in vitro* hepatoprotective activity assay

In vivo Activity Assay

In vivo testing involves experimental animals as models. Hepatotoxicity is generated in animal models by administering known doses of hepatotoxins such as CCl_4, paracetamol, ethanol, *etc*. Plant extracts suspected of having a hepatoprotective effect can be given simultaneously or after the administration of chemical inducers, and then several levels of biomarkers of liver damage can be measured. Histopathology of liver tissue can also be observed to see the level of repair in the tissue and assigned the effect at the molecular, specific proteins or genes expression can be analyzed [87]. The principle of *in vivo* testing is shown in Fig. (**9**), and an example of *in vivo* testing on natural ingredients with a hepatoprotective effect is shown in Table **4**.

Table 4. *In vivo* hepatoprotective activity studies of natural product.

Source	Bioactive compound	Part used	Dose	Animal model, Inducer	Hepatoprotective effects	Ref
Glycyrriza uralensis Fischer	glycyrrhizic acid, liquiritin, and liquiritigenin,	Root, 70% ethanolic extract	100 mg/kg	Male C57BL/6 mice, ethanol	↓AST, ↓ ALT, ↑GSH, ↓TNFα	[18]
Sweet orange (*Citrus sinensis*)	n.d.	Peel, water extract	10 and 100 mg/kg BW for 28 days	Male Wistar rats, CCl_4	↓AST & ALT level, improving the histological architecture of the rat, ↑GSH, ↑ SOD activity, ↑ GPx activity, ↑CYP2E1 activity,	[97]
Brassica rapa var. rapa L	sinapine thiocyanate	Seed, water extract and ethanolic extract	600 mg/kg	Male Kunming mice, CCl_4	↓ ALT and AST, ↑SOD activity, exhibited a marked improvement in the liver histopathology	[98]
Red ginseng (*Panax ginseng* Meyer)	Ginsenoside Rg3 G-Rg3	Not mentioned	5 or 10 mg/kg and totally for 4 weeks	Male-specific pathogen-free (SPF) ICR mice, thioacetamide (TAA)	↓ ALT and AST, ↓LPO, activate PI3K/Akt-signaling cascade	[99]
Panax ginseng Mayer	ginsenoside-Rg2 (G-Rg2) and -Rh1 (G-Rh1)	Not mentioned	20 mg/kg	ICR mice (female), lipopolysaccharide (LPS)	protected liver damage (liver histopathology) ↑ Nrf2 expression, ↓ CD45 expression	[15]
Polygonum cuspidatum, mulberries, peanuts, grape and red wine	Resveratrol	Not mentioned	0,1-0,6 g/kg	tilapia (*Oreochromisniloticus*), H_2O_2	Resveratrol 0.6 g/kg diet for 60 days significantly ameliorated H_2O_2-induced liver injury	[100]

(Table 4) cont.....

Source	Bioactive compound	Part used	Dose	Animal model, Inducer	Hepatoprotective effects	Ref
Vitis vinifera	Resveratrol	Not mentioned	(250 mg/kg BW/day	female Wistar rats with alcoholic liver disease (ALD)	↓ AST and ALT, ↑ hepatic antioxidant enzymes, ↓ inflammation-related genes (CYP2E1, FasL, and TNF-□) expression, ↓oxidative stress, ↓cleaved caspase 3 activity (apoptosis), ↓oxidative stress and inflammation.	[101]
Vitis vinifera	Resveratrol	Not mentioned	10 mg/kg	male Sprague-Dawley rats	↓cleaved caspase-3 and MDA levels, ↑GSH levels.	[102]
Morinda citrifolia (Noni)	n.d.	Fruit, water extract (juice)	20% w/v, 7 days	female Sprague-Dawley (SD) rats, CCl4	Supress ALT (50%) and AST (68%) compared to placebo	[20]
Morinda citrifolia (Noni)	*flavanoids (rutin, quercetin, and kaempferol)	Leaf, methanolic extract	500-1000 mg/kg	Ovariectomized female Sprague Dawley rats	↑ SOD and GPx,) level, ↑ ALP, ↓ liver lipids infiltration, prevent mitochondrial damage, maintain the normal liver histology and ultrastructure	[103]
Sea cucumber (*Holothuria atra*)	*chlorogenic acid (92.86%), pyrogallol (2.99%), rutin (1.83%), coumaric acid (1.55%)	Solvent for extraction: acetonitrile and 0.1% trifluoroacetic acid at a proportion of 60:40 (v/v)	14.4 mg/kg, 8 weeks	Female Swiss albino rats, thioacetamide (TAA)	↓direct bilirubin, ↓AST, ↓ALT, ↓MDA, ↓serum γ-globulin, ↑ SOD and GPx activities,	[104]
Acanthopleura vaillantii (Chiton)	*Flavidin (26,4), Zeaxanthine (16,48%)		10-20 mg/kg BB	male Swiss Albino, CCl₄	↑GSH, ↑ SOD, ↑albumin content, ↓ALT, ↓AST, reduced hepatic fibrosis	[104]
Zizyphus jujube cv. Shaanbeitanzao	*heteropolysaccharides: L-arabinose (50.2%), d-galactose (16.5%), d-galacturonic acid (10.9%)	Fruit pulp, water extract	400 extract mg/kg	kunming male mice, CCl₄	↓ALT, ↓AST, ↓MDA, ↓LDH,	[27]
Berberis vulgaris L	Berberine	Bark, ethanolic extract	50 mg/kg	male Swiss mice, CCl₄	Pretreatment: ↓ 50% ALT, ↓ AST, ↓ bilirubin	[105]
Musa paradisiaca	n.d.	Stem, alcoholic and aqueous extract	250-500 mg/kg	Male and female rats, CCl₄& paracetamol	↓SGOT, ↓SGPT, ↓ALP, ↓bilirubin, protected liver damage (liver histopathology)	[106]

(Table 4) cont.....

Source	Bioactive compound	Part used	Dose	Animal model, Inducer	Hepatoprotective effects	Ref
Phyllanthus niruri	Corilagin, isocorilagin, kaempferolrhamnoside, brevifolin carboxylic acid	aerial parts, 50%, 70% and 80% ethanolic extract	25-200 mg/kg	Male Wistar rats, CCl_4	↓AST, ↓ALT, ↓ALP, ↓LDH, ↓total cholesterol (TC), ↓triglycyrides (TG), ↓total bilirubin (TB), ↓glucose, ↓total proteins (TP), ↓urea, ↓creatinine, ↓TNF-α, NF-KB, IL-6, IL-8, IL10 and COX-2 expression, ↑SOD, ↑CAT, ↑GR, ↑GPx maintain the normal liver histology	[95]
Swertiamus sotii	Swertiamarin	Not mentioned	100-200 mg/kg	Male Sprague-Dawley, CCl_4	↓ALT, ↓AST, ↓ALP, ↓MDA, ↑SOD, ↑GPx, ↑GSH, ↓ inflammatory cytokines/ chemokines (iNOS, IL-1β), ↑ CYPs, ↑PDZK1, up-regulated the expression of Nrf2, HO-1 and NQO1 compared with the CCl4 group.	[107]
Garcinia mangostana	α-mangostin	Not mentioned	12.5-25 mg/kg, 7 days	Adult male ICR mice, lipopolysaccharide/D-galactosamine	↓MDA, ↓ALT, ↓AST, ↓TNF-α, ↓IL-1β, IL-6, ↑GSH, ↑SOD, ↑CAT, ↑Nrf2, ↓TLR4	[108]
Mangifera indica	mangiferin	Not mentioned	5-20 mg/kg	Male BALB/c mice, lipopolysaccharide/D-galactosamine	↓ALT, ↓AST, ↓IL-1β, ↓TNF-α, ↓MCP-1, ↓RANTES, ↓MDA, ↓ROS, ↑ Nrf2,↓NLRP3, ↓ASC, ↓caspase-1, ↓IL-1β, ↓TNF-α	[109]
Mangifera indica		Leaf, water extract		male Wistar rats		
Moringa oleifera	*quercetin, gallic acid and caffeic acid	aerial parts, methanolic extract	2% and 4% (extract powder)	Adult male Wistar rats,	↓ALT, ↓AST	[110]
Daniella oliveri	*rutin, narcissin and quercetin	stem bark, ethanolic extract	200 extract mg/kg	Male albino Wistar rats, CCl_4	↓AST, ↓ALT, ↓ALP, ↓GGT, ↓ bilirubin, ↑GSH, ↑SOD, ↑CAT, ↑GPx	[111]
Ammi majus	n.d.	Seed, alcoholic extract	4-16 mg/rat	Male and female albino rats, CCl_4	↓AST, ↓ALT, ↓ALP, ↓bilirubin, ↓MDA, ↑GSH	[1]

(Table 4) cont.....

Source	Bioactive compound	Part used	Dose	Animal model, Inducer	Hepatoprotective effects	Ref
Bathysa cuspidata	n.d.	Bark	200-400 mg/kg	Male Wistar rats, CCl_4	↓AST, ↓ALT, ↓GGT, ↑SOD,↑CAT, reduction in lipid droplets and necrosis in the liver	[112]
Hancornia speciosa	*Chlorogenic acid, rutin	Fruit, water extract	200 mg extract /Kg	Female Wistar rat, Acetaminophen	↓AST, ↓ALT, ↓GGT, ↓MDA, ↑SOD, ↓hepatocellular degeneration	[91]
Terminalia chebula	chebulinic acid	Fruit, gradient extraction	37.5, 75 and 150 mg/kg	Male ICR mice, CCl_4	↓AST, ↓ALT, ↓MDA, ↑SOD, ↑Nrf2, HO-1, ↓ liver injury in histology evaluation	[92]
Citrus aurantium	*Nobiletin and tangeretin,	Peel, ethanolic extract	50-200 mg/kg	Male C57BL/6 mice,	↓AST, ↓ALT, ↓MDA, ↑GSH,↑SOD, ↑Nrf2, ↑HO-1, ↓IL-family, ↓TNF-α.	[113]
Citrus sinensis L	n.d.	Peel, water extract	Water extract 10 & 100 mg/kg, Hesperidin: 0.1 mg/kg	Male Wistar rats, CCl_4	↓AST, ↓ALT,↓TBARS (MDA), ↑SOD, ↑GPx, ↑CAT, recover the hepatocytes from necrosis. Note: HD at 0.1 mg/kg bw did not sustain any protective effect against oxidative stress induced by CCl4	[97]
*Acanthus ilicifolius*L	n.d.	Leaf, ethanolic extract	250 mg and 500 mg/kg	Male Wistar rats, CCl_4	↓AST, ↓ALT, ↓ALP both in serum and tissue	[114]
Garcinia mangostana	n.d	Peel, ethanolic extract	250 mg and 500 mg/kg	Male Sprague Dawley rats, TAA	↓AST, ↓ALT, ↓ALP, ↓MDA, ↓bilirubin, ↑SOD, ↑CAT	[115]
Phyllanthus amarus	phyllanthin	Aerial parts, gradient extraction	10 mg/kg	Female Swiss mice, CCl_4	↓AST, ↓ALT, ↑CAT, ↑SOD, ↓LPO, ↑GPx, ↑GR, ↑GST, restore the normal architecture and arrangement of hepatocytes	[66]
Garcinia mangostana	α-mangostin	Peel	25 mg/day	Sprague Dawley (SD) rats,high fat diet	↓TBARS (MDA), ↓ROS, ↑SOD, ↑GSH, ↑GPx, ↑GR, ↑CAT, ↑mitochondrial functionality, ↓caspases 9 and 3,	[116]

(Table 4) cont.....

Source	Bioactive compound	Part used	Dose	Animal model, Inducer	Hepatoprotective effects	Ref
Withania somnifera	withanolide	Root, methanolic extract	50, 100 and 200mg/kg	Male Wistar rats, acetaminophen	↓AST, ↓ALT, ↓ALP, ↓bilirubin, ↓TNF-α, ↓IL-1β, ↓iNOS, ↓COX-II mRNA expression	[117]
Andrographis paniculata	*Andrographolide, andrographiside, neoandrographolide	Leaf	100 mg/kg	Male Swiss mice, CCl₄/ tBHP	↓ALT, ↓ALP, ↓MDA, ↑GSH,	[118]

* = major identified compound, the activity not directly tested

n.d. = not determine

Clinical Study

Individuals with severe hepatitis B were randomly assigned to a matrine therapy group (n=60) or a placebo control group (n=60) for a total of 120 patients. The matrine group patients were administered 100 mg of matrine per day for 90 days intramuscularly (an alkaloid derived from the traditional Chinese herb of Radix SophoraeFlavescentis, Guangzhou, Guangzhou, China). In terms of recovery of clinical symptoms and indicators, liver function recovery, and serum conversion from HBe antigen to HBe antibody, as well as from positive to negative serum HBV DNA, substantial variations were observed between both the two groups of patients [119]. IFN-resistant chronic hepatitis C patients with aminotransferase levels twice or more than normal were treated with glycyrrhizin injectable therapy, which reduced the incidence of hepatocellular cancer by a significant amount [120]. An example of a clinical study on natural ingredients with a hepatoprotective effect is shown in Table **5**.

Table 5. Clinical study of hepatoprotective activity studies of natural product.

Source	Bioactive compound	Dose	Subject	Method	Result	Ref
Hordeum vulgare L. (Barley)	*Saponarin	480 mg/day, 12 weeks	Total=76 (habitual alcohol drinkers),	randomized, double-blinded, placebo-controlled trial.	↓liver enzyme, ↑glutathione-s-transferase	[121]
Cynara scolymus L (Artichoke)	n.d.	600 mg/day, 2-month	Total=99 (Non-alcoholic fatty liver disease (NFLD) patients), Treatment=49	randomized double-blind placebo-controlled trial.	↓ALT, ↓AST, ↑ AST/ALT ratio, ↓total bilirubin. Doppler sonography showed increased hepatic vein flow	[122]

(Table 5) cont.....

Source	Bioactive compound	Dose	Subject	Method	Result	Ref
Silybum marianum	silymarin	700 mg/ 3 times daily, 48 weeks	Total=99 (Nonalcoholic Steatohepatitis (NASH) patients), Treatment=49	randomized, double-blind, placebo-controlled trial	Do not reduce NAS score ≥30%, ↓fibrosis (based on histology)	[123]
Silybum marianum	silymarin	420 and 700-mg/3 times daily, 24 weeks	154 (Chronic Hepatitis C Patients Unsuccessfully Treated With Interferon Therapy)	Multicenter, double-blind, placebo-controlled trial	Higher than customary doses of silymarin do not significantly reduce serum ALT.	[124]
Ganoderma lucidum	n.d.	225 mg/day, 6 months	42 (healthy volunteer), treatment=21	Randomized crossover clinical trial	↓AST, ↓ALT, ↓GGT, ↓TBARS, ↑GSH	[125]
Glycyrrhiza glabra (liquorice)	Glycyrrhizin	Not mentioned, 12 days	12 (habitual alcohol drinkers), treatment=6	Randomized, double-blind, placebo-controlled, crossover study	administration glycyrrhizin give no significant increases in liver function enzyme (ALT, AST, GGT, ALP) compared to control	[82]
Antrodia cinnamomea Mycelium	Antrodin A, Antrodin C, 4-Acetylantroquinonol B	420 mg mg/3 times daily, 6 months	Total=42 (Nonalcoholic Steatohepatitis (NASH) patients), treatment=21	Randomized, Double-Blind, Placebo-Controlled Trial	↓ pro-inflammatory cytokines ↓ clinical severity ↓Hepatic Steatosis Grade	[126]

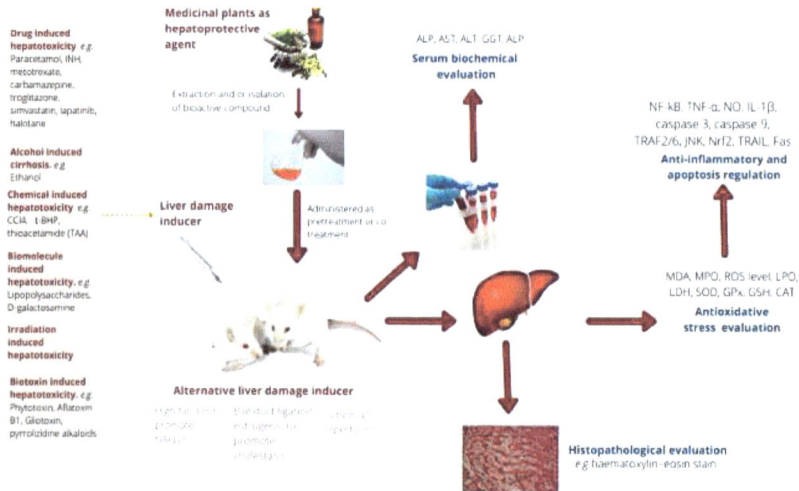

Fig. (9). Common metod of *In vivo* hepatoprotective activity assay

CONCLUDING REMARKS

Hepatoprotective agents can be obtained by utilizing natural materials or plants that are around us. These plants are *Silybum marianum, Moringa oleifera, Garcinia mangostana, Glycyrrhiza glabra, Mangifera indica, Amaranthus spinosus, Andrographis paniculata, Phyllanthus* species (*amarus, niruri, emblica*), *Curcuma* species (*longa, xanthorrhiza, manganese*), and *Citrus species sinensis, unshiu, grandis*) which have been widely used for the treatment of liver disease. The plant contains active compounds that are effective in protecting the day such as chlorogenic acid, curcumin, quercetin, hesperidin, rutin, betalains, apigenin, sylimarin, phyllanthin, mangiferin, -mangostin, bellidifoline, ginsenosides, glycyrrhizin, lycopene, and andrographolide.

REFERENCES

[1]   Mutlag, S.H.; Ismael, D.K.; Al-shawi, N.N. Study the possible hepatoprotective effect of different doses of *Ammi majus* seed's extract against CCl$_4$ induced liver damage in rats. *Int J Compr Pharm,* **2011**, *2*(9), 1-5.

[2]   Park, C.M.; Cha, Y.S.; Youn, H.J.; Cho, C.W.; Song, Y.S. Amelioration of oxidative stress by dandelion extract through CYP2E1 suppression against acute liver injury induced by carbon tetrachloride in sprague-dawley rats. *Phytother. Res.,* **2010**, *24*(9), 1347-1353.
        [http://dx.doi.org/10.1002/ptr.3121] [PMID: 20812277]

[3]   Moreno, M.G.; Reyes, G.G. The role of oxidative stress in thedevelopment of alcoholic liver disease. *Gastroenterol Mex,* **2014**, *79*, 135-144.

[4]   Panjaitan, R.G.P.; Manalu, W.; Handharyani, E. Chairul. Hepatoprotector activity of methanol extract and its derivates fractions of *Eurycomalongifolia* Jack roots. *J. Vet.,* **2011**, *12*, 319-325.

[5]   Sulaimon, LA; Obuotor, EM; Rabiu, LA; Shehu, AA; Aliyu, M; Shiro, MQ Antioxidant and hepatoprotectivepetentials of ethanol stem bark extract of Daniella oliveri (rolfe) hutch and dalz (*Caesalpinaceae*). *Synergy,* **2020**, *11*, 100067.

[6]   Sudjarwo, S.A.; Wardani, G.; Farida, N.; Andayani, R.; Kuntoro, M. The potency of red seaweed (*Eucheuma cottonii*) extracts as hepatoprotector on lead acetate-induced hepatotoxicity in mice. *Pharmacognosy Res.,* **2017**, *9*(3), 282-286.
        [http://dx.doi.org/10.4103/pr.pr_69_16] [PMID: 28827971]

[7]   Farzaei, M.; Zobeiri, M.; Parvizi, F.; El-Senduny, F.; Marmouzi, I.; Coy-Barrera, E.; Naseri, R.; Nabavi, S.; Rahimi, R.; Abdollahi, M. Curcumin in liver diseases: A systematic review of the cellular mechanisms of oxidative stress and clinical perspective. *Nutrients,* **2018**, *10*(7), 855.
        [http://dx.doi.org/10.3390/nu10070855] [PMID: 29966389]

[8]   Karthivashan, G.; Arulselvan, P.; Fakurazi, S. Pathways involved in acetaminophen hepatotoxicity with specific targets for inhibition/downregulation. *RSC Advances,* **2015**, *5*(76), 62040-62051.
        [http://dx.doi.org/10.1039/C5RA07838E]

[9]   Paoletti, F.; Mocali, A. Determination of superoxide dismutase activity by purely chemical system based on NAD(P)H oOxidation. *Methods Enzymol.,* **1990**, *186*, 209-220.
        [http://dx.doi.org/10.1016/0076-6879(90)86110-H] [PMID: 2233293]

[10]   Fernández-Checa, J.C.; Kaplowitz, N.; García-Ruiz, C.; Colell, A.; Miranda, M.; Marí, M.; Ardite, E.; Morales, A. GSH transport in mitochondria: Defense against TNF-induced oxidative stress and alcohol-induced defect. *Am. J. Physiol.,* **1997**, *273*(1 Pt 1), G7-G17.
        [PMID: 9252504]

[11] Rajopadhye, A.; Upadhye, A.S. Estimation of bioactive compound, maslinic acid by HPTLC, and evaluation of hepatoprotective activity on fruit pulp of Ziziphus jujuba Mill. cultivars in India. Evid-Based Compl Alt Med, **2016**; pp. 1-8.

[12] Kang, T.C. Nuclear factor-erythroid 2-related factor 2 (nrf2) and mitochondrial dynamics/mitophagy in neurological diseases. *Antioxidants,* **2020**, *9*(7), 617.
[http://dx.doi.org/10.3390/antiox9070617] [PMID: 32679689]

[13] Ma, Q. Role of nrf2 in oxidative stress and toxicity. *Annu. Rev. Pharmacol. Toxicol.,* **2013**, *53*(1), 401-426.
[http://dx.doi.org/10.1146/annurev-pharmtox-011112-140320] [PMID: 23294312]

[14] Chen, Z.; Tian, R.; She, Z.; Cai, J.; Li, H. Role of oxidative stress in the pathogenesis of nonalcoholic fatty liver disease. *Free Radic. Biol. Med.,* **2020**, *152*, 116-141.
[http://dx.doi.org/10.1016/j.freeradbiomed.2020.02.025] [PMID: 32156524]

[15] Nguyen, T.L.L.; Huynh, D.T.N.; Jin, Y.; Jeon, H.; Heo, K.S. Protective effects of ginsenoside-Rg2 and -Rh1 on liver function through inhibiting TAK1 and STAT3-mediated inflammatory activity and Nrf2/ARE-mediated antioxidant signaling pathway. *Arch. Pharm. Res.,* **2021**, *44*(2), 241-252.
[http://dx.doi.org/10.1007/s12272-020-01304-4] [PMID: 33537886]

[16] Huynh, D.T.N.; Jin, Y.; Myung, C.S.; Heo, K.S. Inhibition of p90RSK is critical to abolish Angiotensin II-induced rat aortic smooth muscle cell proliferation and migration. *Biochem. Biophys. Res. Commun.,* **2020**, *523*(1), 267-273.
[http://dx.doi.org/10.1016/j.bbrc.2019.12.053] [PMID: 31864701]

[17] Irie, T.; Muta, T.; Takeshige, K. TAK1 mediates an activation signal from toll-like receptor(s) to nuclear factor-κB in lipopolysaccharide-stimulated macrophages. *FEBS Lett.,* **2000**, *467*(2-3), 160-164.
[http://dx.doi.org/10.1016/S0014-5793(00)01146-7] [PMID: 10675530]

[18] Jung, J.C.; Lee, Y.H.; Kim, S.H.; Kim, K.J.; Kim, K.M.; Oh, S.; Jung, Y.S. Hepatoprotective effect of licorice, the root of *Glycyrrhiza uralensis* Fischer, in alcohol-induced fatty liver disease. *BMC Complement. Altern. Med.,* **2015**, *16*(1), 19.
[http://dx.doi.org/10.1186/s12906-016-0997-0] [PMID: 26801973]

[19] Arteel, G.E. Oxidants and antioxidants in alcohol-induced liver disease. *Gastroenterology,* **2003**, *124*(3), 778-790.
[http://dx.doi.org/10.1053/gast.2003.50087] [PMID: 12612915]

[20] Wang, M.Y.; Nowicki, D.; Anderson, G.; Jensen, J.; West, B. Liver protective effects of *Morinda citrifolia* (Noni). *Plant Foods Hum. Nutr.,* **2008**, *63*(2), 59-63.
[http://dx.doi.org/10.1007/s11130-008-0070-3] [PMID: 18317933]

[21] Cao, L.; Quan, X.B.; Zeng, W.J.; Yang, X.O.; Wang, M.J. Mechanism of hepatocyte apoptosis. *J. Cell Death,* **2016**, *9*, JCD.S39824.
[http://dx.doi.org/10.4137/JCD.S39824] [PMID: 28058033]

[22] Malhi, H.; Gores, G.J. Cellular and molecular mechanisms of liver injury. *Gastroenterology,* **2008**, *134*(6), 1641-1654.
[http://dx.doi.org/10.1053/j.gastro.2008.03.002] [PMID: 18471544]

[23] Shanmugarajan, T.S.; Prithwish, N.; Somasundaram, I.; Arunsundar, M.; Niladri, M.; Lavande, J.P.; Ravichandiran, V. Mitigation of azathioprine-induced oxidative hepatic injury by the flavonoid quercetin in wistar rats. *Toxicol. Mech. Methods,* **2008**, *18*(8), 653-660.
[http://dx.doi.org/10.1080/15376510802205791] [PMID: 20020851]

[24] Chandan, B.K.; Saxena, A.K.; Shukla, S.; Sharma, N.; Gupta, D.K.; Suri, K.A.; Suri, J.; Bhadauria, M.; Singh, B. Hepatoprotective potential of *Aloe barbadens* Mill. against carbon tetrachloride induced hepatotoxicity. *J. Ethnopharmacol.,* **2007**, *111*(3), 560-566.
[http://dx.doi.org/10.1016/j.jep.2007.01.008] [PMID: 17291700]

[25] Shaker, E.; Mahmoud, H.; Mnaa, S. Silymarin, the antioxidant component and *Silybum marianum* extracts prevent liver damage. *Food Chem. Toxicol.,* **2010**, *48*(3), 803-806.
[http://dx.doi.org/10.1016/j.fct.2009.12.011] [PMID: 20034535]

[26] Xu, L.; Gao, J.; Wang, Y.; Yu, W.; Zhao, X.; Yang, X. Myrica rubra extracts protect the liver from CCl₄-induced damage. *Evid-Based Compl Alt Med,* **2011**, *2011*

[27] Saha, P.; Talukdar, A.D.; Nath, R.; Sarker, S.D.; Nahar, L.; Sahu, J.; Choudhury, M.D. Role of natural phenolics in hepatoprotection: A mechanistic review and analysis of regulatory network of associated genes. *Front. Pharmacol.,* **2019**, *10*(5), 509.
[http://dx.doi.org/10.3389/fphar.2019.00509] [PMID: 31178720]

[28] Wang, D.; Zhao, Y.; Jiao, Y.; Yu, L.; Yang, S.; Yang, X. Antioxidative and hepatoprotective effects of the polysaccharides from *Ziziphus jujube* cv. Shaanbeitanzao. *Carbohydr. Polym.,* **2012**, *88*(4), 1453-1459.
[http://dx.doi.org/10.1016/j.carbpol.2012.02.046]

[29] Kasai, H.; Fukada, S.; Yamaizumi, Z.; Sugie, S.; Mori, H. Action of chlorogenic acid in vegetables and fruits as an inhibitor of 8-hydroxydeoxyguanosine formation *in vitro* and in a rat carcinogenesis model. *Food Chem. Toxicol.,* **2000**, *38*(5), 467-471.
[http://dx.doi.org/10.1016/S0278-6915(00)00014-4] [PMID: 10762733]

[30] Yun, N.; Kang, J.W.; Lee, S.M. Protective effects of chlorogenic acid against ischemia/reperfusion injury in rat liver: Molecular evidence of its antioxidant and anti-inflammatory properties. *J. Nutr. Biochem.,* **2012**, *23*(10), 1249-1255.
[http://dx.doi.org/10.1016/j.jnutbio.2011.06.018] [PMID: 22209001]

[31] Shi, H.; Dong, L.; Dang, X.; Liu, Y.; Jiang, J.; Wang, Y.; Lu, X.; Guo, X. Effect of chlorogenic acid on LPS-induced proinflammatory signaling in hepatic stellate cells. *Inflamm. Res.,* **2013**, *62*(6), 581-587.
[http://dx.doi.org/10.1007/s00011-013-0610-7] [PMID: 23483217]

[32] Zhenlong, C.; Yuhui, Y.; Shumei, M.; Qingsheng, F.; Xiaoming, S.; Baichuan, D. Hepatoprotective effect of chlorogenic acid against chronic liver injury in inflammatory rats. *J. Funct. Foods,* **2019**, *62*(103540), 1-13.

[33] Naveed, M.; Hejazi, V.; Abbas, M.; Kamboh, A.A.; Khan, G.J.; Shumzaid, M.; Ahmad, F.; Babazadeh, D.; FangFang, X.; Modarresi-Ghazani, F.; WenHua, L.; XiaoHui, Z. Chlorogenic acid (CGA): A pharmacological review and call for further research. *Biomed. Pharmacother.,* **2018**, *97*, 67-74.
[http://dx.doi.org/10.1016/j.biopha.2017.10.064] [PMID: 29080460]

[34] AlGamdi, N.; Mullen, W.; Crozier, A. Tea prepared from *Anastatica hirerochuntica* seeds contains a diversity of antioxidant flavonoids, chlorogenic acids and phenolic compounds. *Phytochemistry,* **2011**, *72*(2-3), 248-254.
[http://dx.doi.org/10.1016/j.phytochem.2010.11.017] [PMID: 21176927]

[35] Romero-González, R.R.; Verpoorte, R. Salting-out gradients in centrifugal partition chromatography for the isolation of chlorogenic acids from green coffee beans. *J. Chromatogr. A,* **2009**, *1216*(19), 4245-4251.
[http://dx.doi.org/10.1016/j.chroma.2009.02.007] [PMID: 19233365]

[36] Tajik, N.; Tajik, M.; Mack, I.; Enck, P. The potential effects of chlorogenic acid, the main phenolic components in coffee, on health: A comprehensive review of the literature. *Eur. J. Nutr.,* **2017**, *56*(7), 2215-2244.
[http://dx.doi.org/10.1007/s00394-017-1379-1] [PMID: 28391515]

[37] Fahmy, T.A.; Nahla, S.H.; Rehab, R.A. Hepatoprotective and antiproliferative activity of moringinine, chlorogenic acid and quercetin. *Int J Res Med Sci,* **2016**, *4*(4), 1147-1153.

[38]   Suphachai, C. Antioxidant and anticancer activities of *Moringa oleifera* leaves. *J. Med. Plants Res.,*
         2014, *8*(7), 318-325.
         [http://dx.doi.org/10.5897/JMPR2013.5353]

[39]   Plazas, M.; Andújar, I.; Vilanova, S.; Hurtado, M.; Gramazio, P.; Herraiz, F.J.; Prohens, J. Breeding
         for chlorogenic acid content in eggplant: Interest and prospects. *Not. Bot. Horti Agrobot. Cluj-Napoca,*
         2013, *41*(1), 26-35.
         [http://dx.doi.org/10.15835/nbha4119036]

[40]   Li, G.; Chen, J.B.; Wang, C.; Xu, Z.; Nie, H.; Qin, X.Y.; Chen, X.M.; Gong, Q. Curcumin protects
         against acetaminophen-induced apoptosis in hepatic injury. *World J. Gastroenterol.,* **2013**, *19*(42),
         7440-7446.
         [http://dx.doi.org/10.3748/wjg.v19.i42.7440] [PMID: 24259976]

[41]   Lee, G.H.; Lee, H.Y.; Choi, M.K.; Chung, H.W.; Kim, S.W.; Chae, H.J. Protective effect of *Curcuma
         longa* L. extract on CCl$_4$-induced acute hepatic stress. *BMC Res. Notes,* **2017**, *10*(1), 77.
         [http://dx.doi.org/10.1186/s13104-017-2409-z] [PMID: 28057050]

[42]   Hemeida, R.A.M.; Mohafez, O.M. Curcumin attenuates methotraxate-induced hepatic oxidative
         damage in rats. *J. Egypt. Natl. Canc. Inst.,* **2008**, *20*(2), 141-148.
         [PMID: 20029470]

[43]   Hashish, E.A.; Elgaml, S.A. Hepatoprotective and nephroprotective effect of curcumin against copper
         toxicity in rats. *Indian J. Clin. Biochem.,* **2016**, *31*(3), 270-277.
         [http://dx.doi.org/10.1007/s12291-015-0527-8] [PMID: 27382197]

[44]   Kaur, G.; Tirkey, N.; Bharrhan, S.; Chanana, V.; Rishi, P.; Chopra, K. Inhibition of oxidative stress
         and cytokine activity by curcumin in amelioration of endotoxin-induced experimental hepatoxicity in
         rodents. *Clin. Exp. Immunol.,* **2006**, *145*(2), 313-321.
         [http://dx.doi.org/10.1111/j.1365-2249.2006.03108.x] [PMID: 16879252]

[45]   Salama, S.M.; Abdulla, M.A.; AlRashdi, A.S.; Ismail, S.; Alkiyumi, S.S.; Golbabapour, S.
         Hepatoprotective effect of ethanolic extract of *Curcuma longa* on thioacetamide induced liver cirrhosis
         in rats. *BMC Complement. Altern. Med.,* **2013**, *13*(1), 56.
         [http://dx.doi.org/10.1186/1472-6882-13-56] [PMID: 23496995]

[46]   Amália, P.M.; Possa, M.N.; Augusto, M.C.; Francisca, L.S. Quercetin prevents oxidative stress in
         cirrhotic rats. *Dig. Dis. Sci.,* **2007**, *52*(10), 2616-2621.
         [http://dx.doi.org/10.1007/s10620-007-9748-x] [PMID: 17431769]

[47]   Padma, V.V.; Baskaran, R.; Roopesh, R.S.; Poornima, P. Quercetin attenuates lindane induced
         oxidative stress in wistar rats. *Mol. Biol. Rep.,* **2012**, *39*(6), 6895-6905.
         [http://dx.doi.org/10.1007/s11033-012-1516-0] [PMID: 22302394]

[48]   Wu, L.; Wang, C.; Li, J.; Li, S.; Feng, J.; Liu, T.; Xu, S.; Wang, W.; Lu, X.; Chen, K.; Xia, Y.; Fan,
         X.; Guo, C. Hepatoprotective effect of quercetin *via* TRAF6/JNK pathway in acute hepatitis. *Biomed.
         Pharmacother.,* **2017**, *96*, 1137-1146.
         [http://dx.doi.org/10.1016/j.biopha.2017.11.109] [PMID: 29174851]

[49]   Tabeshpour, J.; Hosseinzadeh, H.; Hashemzaei, M.; Karimi, G. A review of the hepatoprotective
         effects of hesperidin, a flavanon glycoside in citrus fruits, against natural and chemical toxicities.
         Daru, **2020**, *28*(1), 305-317.
         [http://dx.doi.org/10.1007/s40199-020-00344-x] [PMID: 32277430]

[50]   Tirkey, N.; Pilkhwal, S.; Kuhad, A.; Chopra, K. Hasperidin, a citrus bioflavonoid, decreases the
         oxidative stress produced by carbon tetrachloride in rat liver and kidney. *BMC Pharmacol.,* **2005**, *5*(1),
         2.
         [http://dx.doi.org/10.1186/1471-2210-5-2]

[51] Kaur, G.; Tirkey, N.; Chopra, K. Beneficial effect of hesperidin on lipopolysaccharide-induced hepatotoxicity. *Toxicology,* **2006**, *226*(2-3), 152-160.
[http://dx.doi.org/10.1016/j.tox.2006.06.018] [PMID: 16919860]

[52] Pires Das Neves, R.N.; Carvalho, F.; Carvalho, M.; Fernandes, E.; Soares, E.; Bastos, M.D.L.; Pereira, M.D.L. Protective activity of hesperidin and lipoic acid against sodium arsenite acute toxicity in mice. *Toxicol. Pathol.,* **2004**, *32*(5), 527-535.
[http://dx.doi.org/10.1080/01926230490502566] [PMID: 15603538]

[53] Khan, R.A.; Khan, M.R.; Sahreen, S. CCl_4-induced hepatotoxicity: protective effect of rutin on p53, CYP2E1 and the antioxidative status in rat. *BMC Complement. Altern. Med.,* **2012**, *12*(1), 178.
[http://dx.doi.org/10.1186/1472-6882-12-178] [PMID: 23043521]

[54] Kanika, P.; Dinesh, K.P. Bioactive food as dietary interventions for arthritis and related inflammatory diseases. In: *In the chapter of The beneficial role of rutin, A naturally occurring flavonoid in health promotion and disease prevention: A systematic review and update,* 2nd; Elsevier, **2019**.

[55] Atanassova, M.; Bagdassarian, V. Rutin content in plant products. *J Univ Chem Technol Metallurgy,* **2009**, *44*(2), 201-203.

[56] Gliszczyńska-Świgło, A.; Szymusiak, H.; Malinowska, P. Betanin, the main pigment of red beet: Molecular origin of its exceptionally high free radical-scavenging activity. *Food Addit. Contam.,* **2006**, *23*(11), 1079-1087.
[http://dx.doi.org/10.1080/02652030600986032] [PMID: 17071510]

[57] Albasher, G.; Almeer, R.; Al-Otibi, F.O.; Al-Kubaisi, N.; Mahmoud, A.M. Ameliorative effect of *Beta vulgaris* root extract on chlorpyrifos-induced oxidative stress, inflammation and liver injury in rats. *Biomolecules,* **2019**, *9*(7), 261.
[http://dx.doi.org/10.3390/biom9070261] [PMID: 31284640]

[58] Han, J.; Zhang, Z.; Yang, S.; Wang, J.; Yang, X.; Tan, D. Betanin attenuates paraquat-induced liver toxicity through a mitochondrial pathway. *Food Chem. Toxicol.,* **2014**, *70*, 100-106.
[http://dx.doi.org/10.1016/j.fct.2014.04.038] [PMID: 24799198]

[59] Madadi, E.; Mazloum-Ravasan, S.; Yu, J.S.; Ha, J.W.; Hamishehkar, H.; Kim, K.H. Therapeutic application of betalains: A review. *Plants,* **2020**, *9*(9), 1219.
[http://dx.doi.org/10.3390/plants9091219] [PMID: 32957510]

[60] Yue, S.; Xue, N.; Li, H.; Huang, B.; Chen, Z.; Wang, X. Hepatoprotective effect of apigenin against liver injury *via* the non-canonical NF-κB pathway *In vivo* and *in vitro*. *Inflammation,* **2020**, *43*(5), 1634-1648.
[http://dx.doi.org/10.1007/s10753-020-01238-5] [PMID: 32458347]

[61] Ali, F.; Rahul, ; Naz, F.; Jyoti, S.; Siddique, Y.H. Health functionality of apigenin: A review. *Int. J. Food Prop.,* **2017**, *20*(6), 1197-1238.
[http://dx.doi.org/10.1080/10942912.2016.1207188]

[62] Polyak, S.J.; Ferenci, P.; Pawlotsky, J.M. Hepatoprotective and antiviral functions of silymarin components in hepatitis C virus infection. *Hepatology,* **2013**, *57*(3), 1262-1271.
[http://dx.doi.org/10.1002/hep.26179] [PMID: 23213025]

[63] Gillessen, A.; Schmidt, H.H.J. Silymarin as supportive treatment in liver diseases: A narrative review. *Adv. Ther.,* **2020**, *37*(4), 1279-1301.
[http://dx.doi.org/10.1007/s12325-020-01251-y] [PMID: 32065376]

[64] Federico, A.; Dallio, M.; Loguercio, C. Silymarin/Silybin and chronic liver disease: A marriage of many years. *Molecules,* **2017**, *22*(2), 191.
[http://dx.doi.org/10.3390/molecules22020191] [PMID: 28125040]

[65] Chirdchupunseree, H.; Pramyothin, P. Protective activity of phyllanthin in ethanol-treated primary culture of rat hepatocytes. *J. Ethnopharmacol.,* **2010**, *128*(1), 172-176.
[http://dx.doi.org/10.1016/j.jep.2010.01.003] [PMID: 20064596]

[66]   Krithika, R.; Verma, R.J. Ameliorative effects of phyllanthin on carbon tetrachloride-induced hepatic oxidative damage in mice. *Asian Pac. J. Trop. Dis.,* **2014**, *4*(S1), S64-S70.
[http://dx.doi.org/10.1016/S2222-1808(14)60416-3]

[67]   You, Y.; Zhu, F.; Li, Z.; Zhang, L.; Xie, Y.; Chinnathambi, A.; Alahmadi, T.A.; Lu, B. Phyllanthin prevents diethylnitrosamine (DEN) induced liver carcinogenesis in rats and induces apoptotic cell death in HepG2 cells. *Biomed. Pharmacother.,* **2021**, *137*(February), 111335.
[http://dx.doi.org/10.1016/j.biopha.2021.111335] [PMID: 33581648]

[68]   Asadi-Samani, M.; Kafash-Farkhad, N.; Azimi, N.; Fasihi, A.; Alinia-Ahandani, E.; Rafieian-Kopaei, M. Medicinal plants with hepatoprotective activity in Iranian folk medicine. *Asian Pac. J. Trop. Biomed.,* **2015**, *5*(2), 146-157.
[http://dx.doi.org/10.1016/S2221-1691(15)30159-3]

[69]   Zahra, A.A.; Mohammed, A.A.; Mustafa, K.; Hapipah, M.A.; Mahmood, A.A. Gene expression profiling reveals underlying molecular mechanism of hepatoprotective effect of *Phyllanthusniruri* on thioacetamide-induced hepatotoxicity in Sprague Dawley rats. *BMC Complement. Altern. Med.,* **2013**, *13*(160), 1-10.

[70]   Chowdhury, A.; Lu, J.; Zhang, R.; Nabila, J.; Gao, H.; Wan, Z.; Adelusi Temitope, I.; Yin, X.; Sun, Y. Mangiferin ameliorates acetaminophen-induced hepatotoxicity through APAP-Cys and JNK modulation. *Biomed. Pharmacother.,* **2019**, *117*(April), 109097.
[http://dx.doi.org/10.1016/j.biopha.2019.109097] [PMID: 31212128]

[71]   Pardo-Andreu, G.L.; Barrios, M.F.; Curti, C.; Hernández, I.; Merino, N.; Lemus, Y.; Martínez, I.; Riaño, A.; Delgado, R. Protective effects of *Mangifera indica* L extract (Vimang), and its major component mangiferin, on iron-induced oxidative damage to rat serum and liver. *Pharmacol. Res.,* **2008**, *57*(1), 79-86.
[http://dx.doi.org/10.1016/j.phrs.2007.12.004] [PMID: 18243014]

[72]   Imran, M.; Arshad, M.S.; Butt, M.S.; Kwon, J.H.; Arshad, M.U.; Sultan, M.T. Mangiferin: a natural miracle bioactive compound against lifestyle related disorders. *Lipids Health Dis.,* **2017**, *16*(1), 84.
[http://dx.doi.org/10.1186/s12944-017-0449-y] [PMID: 28464819]

[73]   Obolskiy, D.; Pischel, I.; Siriwatanametanon, N.; Heinrich, M. *Garcinia mangostana* L.: A phytochemical and pharmacological review. *Phytother. Res.,* **2009**, *23*(8), 1047-1065.
[http://dx.doi.org/10.1002/ptr.2730] [PMID: 19172667]

[74]   Fu, T.; Wang, S.; Liu, J.; Cai, E.; Li, H.; Li, P.; Zhao, Y. Protective effects of α-mangostin against acetaminophen-induced acute liver injury in mice. *Eur. J. Pharmacol.,* **2018**, *827*, 173-180.
[http://dx.doi.org/10.1016/j.ejphar.2018.03.002] [PMID: 29563064]

[75]   Zheng, X.Y.; Yang, Y.F.; Li, W.; Zhao, X.; Sun, Y.; Sun, H.; Wang, Y.H.; Pu, X.P. Two xanthones from *Swertia punicea* with hepatoprotective activities *in vitro* and *In vivo*. *J. Ethnopharmacol.,* **2014**, *153*(3), 854-863.
[http://dx.doi.org/10.1016/j.jep.2014.03.058] [PMID: 24690777]

[76]   Xiao, M.H.; Xia, J.Y.; Wang, Z.L.; Hu, W.X.; Fan, Y.L.; Jia, D.Y.; Li, J.; Jing, P.W.; Wang, L.; Wang, Y.P. Ginsenoside Rg1 attenuates liver injury induced by D□galactose in mice. *Exp. Ther. Med.,* **2018**, *16*(5), 4100-4106.
[http://dx.doi.org/10.3892/etm.2018.6727] [PMID: 30402153]

[77]   Ning, C.; Gao, X.; Wang, C.; Huo, X.; Liu, Z.; Sun, H.; Yang, X.; Sun, P.; Ma, X.; Meng, Q.; Liu, K. Hepatoprotective effect of ginsenoside Rg1 from *Panax ginseng* on carbon tetrachloride-induced acute liver injury by activating Nrf2 signaling pathway in mice. *Environ. Toxicol.,* **2018**, *33*(10), 1050-1060.
[http://dx.doi.org/10.1002/tox.22616] [PMID: 29964319]

[78]   Hu, J.N.; Xu, X.Y.; Li, W.; Wang, Y.M.; Liu, Y.; Wang, Z.; Wang, Y.P. Ginsenoside Rk1 ameliorates paracetamol-induced hepatotoxicity in mice through inhibition of inflammation, oxidative stress, nitrative stress and apoptosis. *J. Ginseng Res.,* **2019**, *43*(1), 10-19.
[http://dx.doi.org/10.1016/j.jgr.2017.07.003] [PMID: 30662289]

[79]   Kim, T.W. Ginseng for liver injury: Friend or foe? *Medicines,* **2016**, *3*(4), 33.
       [http://dx.doi.org/10.3390/medicines3040033] [PMID: 28930143]

[80]   Li, J.; Cao, H.; Liu, P.; Cheng, G.; Sun, M. Glycyrrhizic acid in the treatment of liver diseases:
       Literature review. *BioMed Res. Int.,* **2014**, *2014*, 1-15.
       [http://dx.doi.org/10.1155/2014/872139] [PMID: 24963489]

[81]   Tenkerian, C.; El-Sibai, M.; Daher, C.F.; Mroueh, M. Hepatoprotective, antioxidant, and anticancer
       effects of the tragopogon porrifolius methanolic extract. *Evid-Based Complement Altern Med,* **2015**,
       2015

[82]   Chigurupati, H.; Auddy, B.; Biyani, M.; Stohs, S.J. Hepatoprotective effects of a proprietary
       glycyrrhizin product during alcohol consumption: A randomized, double-blind, placebo-controlled,
       crossover study. *Phytother. Res.,* **2016**, *30*(12), 1943-1953.
       [http://dx.doi.org/10.1002/ptr.5699] [PMID: 27539273]

[83]   Jiang, W.; Guo, M.H.; Hai, X. Hepatoprotective and antioxidant effects of lycopene on non-alcoholic
       fatty liver disease in rat. *World J. Gastroenterol.,* **2016**, *22*(46), 10180-10188.
       [http://dx.doi.org/10.3748/wjg.v22.i46.10180] [PMID: 28028366]

[84]   Islam, M.T. Andrographolide, a new hope in the prevention and treatment of metabolic syndrome.
       Front. Pharmacol., **2017**, *8*, 571.
       [http://dx.doi.org/10.3389/fphar.2017.00571] [PMID: 28878680]

[85]   Ye, J.F.; Zhu, H.; Zhou, Z.F.; Xiong, R.B.; Wang, X.W.; Su, L.X.; Luo, B.D. Protective mechanism of
       andrographolide against carbon tetrachloride-induced acute liver injury in mice. *Biol. Pharm. Bull.,*
       2011, *34*(11), 1666-1670.
       [http://dx.doi.org/10.1248/bpb.34.1666] [PMID: 22040877]

[86]   Valvi, A.R.; Mouriya, N.; Athawale, R.B.; Bhatt, N.S. Hepatoprotective Ayurvedic plants :A review.
       J. Complement. Integr. Med., **2016**, *13*(3), 207-215.
       [http://dx.doi.org/10.1515/jcim-2015-0110] [PMID: 27310002]

[87]   Nevzorova, Y.A.; Boyer-Diaz, Z.; Cubero, F.J.; Gracia-Sancho, J. Animal models for liver disease : A
       practical approach for translational research. *J. Hepatol.,* **2020**, *73*(2), 423-440.
       [http://dx.doi.org/10.1016/j.jhep.2020.04.011] [PMID: 32330604]

[88]   Nguyen, T.P.; Tran, C.L.; Vuong, C.H.; Do, T.H.T.; Le, T.D.; Mai, D.T.; Phan, N.M. Flavonoids with
       hepatoprotective activity from the leaves of *Cleome viscosa* L. *Nat. Prod. Res.,* **2017**, *31*(22), 2587-
       2592.
       [http://dx.doi.org/10.1080/14786419.2017.1283497] [PMID: 28135851]

[89]   Tian, D.; Wang, F.; Duan, M.; Cao, L.; Zhang, Y.; Yao, X.; Tang, J. Coumarin analogues from the
       Citrus grandis (L.) Osbeck and their hepatoprotective activity. *J. Agric. Food Chem.,* **2019**, *67*(7),
       1937-1947.
       [http://dx.doi.org/10.1021/acs.jafc.8b06489] [PMID: 30689373]

[90]   Wei, R.; Ma, Q.; Zhong, G.; Su, Y.; Yang, J.; Wang, A. Structural characterization, hepatoprotective
       and antihyperlipidemic activities of alkaloid derivatives from *Murraya koenigii. Phytochem. Lett.,*
       2019, *35*(November), 135-140.

[91]   Santos, R.S.; Chaves-Filho, A.B.; Silva, L.A.S.; Garcia, C.A.D.; Silva, A.R.S.T.; Dolabella, S.S.
       Bioactive compounds and hepatoprotective effect of *Hancornia speciosa* gomes fruit juice on
       acetaminophen-induced hepatotoxicity *In vivo. Nat. Prod. Res.,* **2021**, *22*, 1-5.
       [PMID: 33749461]

[92]   Feng, X.H.; Xu, H.Y.; Wang, J.Y.; Duan, S.; Wang, Y.C.; Ma, C.M. *In vivo* hepatoprotective activity
       and the underlying mechanism of chebulinic acid from *Terminalia chebula* fruit. *Phytomedicine,* **2021**,
       83, 153479.
       [http://dx.doi.org/10.1016/j.phymed.2021.153479] [PMID: 33561764]

[93] Ye, H.; Luo, J.; Hu, D.; Yang, S.; Zhang, A.; Qiu, Y.; Ma, X.; Wang, J.; Hou, J.; Bai, J. Total flavonoids of *Crocus sativus* petals release tert-butyl hydroperoxide-induced oxidative stress in BRL-3A cells. *Oxid. Med. Cell. Longev.,* **2021**, *2021*, 1-15.
[http://dx.doi.org/10.1155/2021/5453047] [PMID: 34194602]

[94] Wang, A.; Liu, Q.; Ye, Y.; Wang, Y.; Lin, L. Identification of hepatoprotective xanthones from the pericarps of *Garcinia mangostana*, guided with tert-butyl hydroperoxide induced oxidative injury in HL-7702 cells. *Food Funct.,* **2015**, *6*(9), 3013-3021.
[http://dx.doi.org/10.1039/C5FO00573F] [PMID: 26189454]

[95] Ezzat, M.I.; Okba, M.M.; Ahmed, S.H.; El-Banna, H.A.; Prince, A.; Mohamed, S.O.; Ezzat, S.M. In-depth hepatoprotective mechanistic study of *Phyllanthus niruri*: *in vitro* and *In vivo* studies and its chemical characterization. *PLoS One,* **2020**, *15*(1), e0226185.
[http://dx.doi.org/10.1371/journal.pone.0226185] [PMID: 31940365]

[96] Wu, J.G.; Kan, Y.J.; Wu, Y.B.; Yi, J.; Chen, T.Q.; Wu, J.Z. Hepatoprotective effect of ganoderma triterpenoids against oxidative damage induced by *tert* -butyl hydroperoxide in human hepatic HepG2 cells. *Pharm. Biol.,* **2016**, *54*(5), 919-929.
[http://dx.doi.org/10.3109/13880209.2015.1091481] [PMID: 26457919]

[97] Chen, S.Y.; Chyau, C.C.; Chu, C.C.; Chen, Y.H.; Chen, T.H.; Duh, P.D. Hepatoprotection using sweet orange peel and its bioactive compound, hesperidin, for CCl$_4$-induced liver injury *In vivo*. *J. Funct. Foods,* **2013**, *5*(4), 1591-1600.
[http://dx.doi.org/10.1016/j.jff.2013.07.001]

[98] Fu, R.; Zhang, Y.; Guo, Y.; Peng, T.; Chen, F. Hepatoprotection using *Brassica rapa* var. rapa L. seeds and its bioactive compound, sinapine thiocyanate, for CCl$_4$-induced liver injury. *J. Funct. Foods,* **2016**, *22*, 73-81.
[http://dx.doi.org/10.1016/j.jff.2016.01.013]

[99] Liu, X.; Mi, X.; Wang, Z.; Zhang, M.; Hou, J.; Jiang, S.; Wang, Y.; Chen, C.; Li, W. Ginsenoside Rg3 promotes regression from hepatic fibrosis through reducing inflammation-mediated autophagy signaling pathway. *Cell Death Dis.,* **2020**, *11*(6), 454.
[http://dx.doi.org/10.1038/s41419-020-2597-7] [PMID: 32532964]

[100] Jia, R.; Li, Y.; Cao, L.; Du, J.; Zheng, T.; Qian, H.; Gu, Z.; Jeney, G.; Xu, P.; Yin, G. Antioxidative, anti-inflammatory and hepatoprotective effects of resveratrol on oxidative stress-induced liver damage in tilapia (Oreochromis niloticus). *Comp. Biochem. Physiol. C Toxicol. Pharmacol.,* **2019**, *215*, 56-66.
[http://dx.doi.org/10.1016/j.cbpc.2018.10.002] [PMID: 30336289]

[101] Peiyuan, H.; Zhiping, H.; Chengjun, S.; Chunqing, W.; Bingqing, L.; Imam, M.U. Resveratrol ameliorates experimental alcoholic liver disease by modulating oxidative stress. *Evid-Based Complement Altern Med,* **2017**, *2017*, 4287890.
[http://dx.doi.org/10.1155/2017/4287890]

[102] Bilen, A.; Mercantepe, F.; Tümkaya, L.; Yilmaz, A.; Batcik, Ş. The hepatoprotective potential of resveratrol in an experimental model of ruptured abdominal aortic aneurysm *via* oxidative stress and apoptosis. *J. Biochem. Mol. Toxicol.,* **2021**, *35*(8), e22836.
[http://dx.doi.org/10.1002/jbt.22836] [PMID: 34075649]

[103] Chong, C.L.G.; Hussan, F.; Othman, F. Hepatoprotective effects of *Morinda citrifolia* leaf extract on ovariectomized rats fed with thermoxidized palm oil diet: Evidence at histological and ultrastructural level. *Oxid. Med. Cell. Longev.,* **2019**, *2019*, 1-10.
[http://dx.doi.org/10.1155/2019/9714302] [PMID: 31827717]

[104] Esmat, A.Y.; Said, M.M.; Soliman, A.A.; El-Masry, K.S.H.; Badiea, E.A. Bioactive compounds, antioxidant potential, and hepatoprotective activity of sea cucumber (*Holothuria atra*) against thioacetamide intoxication in rats. *Nutrition,* **2013**, *29*(1), 258-267.
[http://dx.doi.org/10.1016/j.nut.2012.06.004] [PMID: 23085016]

[105] Hermenean, A.; Popescu, C.; Ardelean, A.; Stan, M.; Hadaruga, N.; Mihali, C.V.; Costache, M.; Dinischiotu, A. Hepatoprotective effects of Berberis vulgaris L. extract/β cyclodextrin on carbon tetrachloride-induced acute toxicity in mice. *Int. J. Mol. Sci.,* **2012**, *13*(7), 9014-9034.
[http://dx.doi.org/10.3390/ijms13079014] [PMID: 22942749]

[106] Nirmala, M.; Girija, K.; Lakshman, K.; Divya, T. Hepatoprotective activity of *Musa paradisiaca* on experimental animal models. *Asian Pac. J. Trop. Biomed.,* **2012**, *2*(1), 11-15.
[http://dx.doi.org/10.1016/S2221-1691(11)60181-0] [PMID: 23569826]

[107] Wu, T.; Li, J.; Li, Y.; Song, H. Antioxidant and hepatoprotective effect of swertiamarin on carbon tetrachloride-induced hepatotoxicity *via* the Nrf2/HO-1 pathway. *Cell. Physiol. Biochem.,* **2017**, *41*(6), 2242-2254.
[http://dx.doi.org/10.1159/000475639] [PMID: 28448964]

[108] Fu, T.; Li, H.; Zhao, Y.; Cai, E.; Zhu, H.; Li, P.; Liu, J. Hepatoprotective effect of α-mangostin against lipopolysaccharide/d-galactosamine-induced acute liver failure in mice. *Biomed. Pharmacother.,* **2018**, *106*(5), 896-901.
[http://dx.doi.org/10.1016/j.biopha.2018.07.034] [PMID: 30119260]

[109] Pan, CW; Pan, ZZ; Hu, JJ; Chen, WL; Zhou, GY; Lin, W. Mangiferin alleviates lipopolysaccharide and D-galactosamine-induced acute liver injury by activating the Nrf2 pathway and inhibiting NLRP3 inflammasome activation. *Eur J Pharmacol,* **2016**, *770*, 85-91.

[110] Asgari-Kafrani, A.; Fazilati, M.; Nazem, H. Hepatoprotective and antioxidant activity of aerial parts of *Moringa oleifera* in prevention of non-alcoholic fatty liver disease in Wistar rats. *S. Afr. J. Bot.,* **2020**, *129*, 82-90.
[http://dx.doi.org/10.1016/j.sajb.2019.01.014]

[111] Sulaimon, L.A.; Obuotor, E.M.; Rabiu, L.A.; Shehu, A.A.; Aliyu, M.; Shiro, M.Q. Antioxidant and hepatoprotective potentials of ethanol stem bark extract of Daniela oliveri (Rolfe) Hutch and Dalz (Caesalpinaceae). *Synergy,* **2020**, *11*, 100067.
[http://dx.doi.org/10.1016/j.synres.2020.100067]

[112] Gonçalves, R.V.; Novaes, R.D.; Leite, J.P.V.; Vilela, E.F.; Cupertino, M.C.; Nunes, L.G.; Matta, S.L.P. Hepatoprotective effect of *Bathysa cuspidata* in a murine model of severe toxic liver injury. *Int. J. Exp. Pathol.,* **2012**, *93*(5), 370-376.
[http://dx.doi.org/10.1111/j.1365-2613.2012.00835.x] [PMID: 22974218]

[113] Choi, B.K.; Kim, T.W.; Lee, D.R.; Jung, W.H.; Lim, J.H.; Jung, J.Y.; Yang, S.H.; Suh, J.W. A polymethoxy flavonoids-rich *Citrus aurantium* extract ameliorates ethanol-induced liver injury through modulation of AMPK and Nrf2-related signals in a binge drinking mouse model. *Phytother. Res.,* **2015**, *29*(10), 1577-1584.
[http://dx.doi.org/10.1002/ptr.5415] [PMID: 26178909]

[114] Babu, B.H.; Shylesh, B.S.; Padikkala, J. Antioxidant and hepatoprotective effect of *Acanthus ilicifolius. Fitoterapia,* **2001**, *72*(3), 272-277.
[http://dx.doi.org/10.1016/S0367-326X(00)00300-2] [PMID: 11295303]

[115] Abood, W.N.; Bradosty, S.W.; Shaikh, F.K.; Salehen, N.A.; Farghadani, R.; Agha, N.F.S.; Al-Medhtiy, M.H.; Kamil, T.D.A.; Agha, A.S.; Abdulla, M.A. *Garcinia mangostana* peel extracts exhibit hepatoprotective activity against thioacetamide-induced liver cirrhosis in rats. *J. Funct. Foods,* **2020**, *74*, 104200.
[http://dx.doi.org/10.1016/j.jff.2020.104200]

[116] Tsai, S.Y.; Chung, P.C.; Owaga, E.E.; Tsai, I.J.; Wang, P.Y.; Tsai, J.I.; Yeh, T.S.; Hsieh, R.H. Alpha-mangostin from mangosteen (*Garcinia mangostana Linn.*) pericarp extract reduces high fat-diet induced hepatic steatosis in rats by regulating mitochondria function and apoptosis. *Nutr. Metab.,* **2016**, *13*(1), 88.
[http://dx.doi.org/10.1186/s12986-016-0148-0] [PMID: 27980597]

[117] Devkar, S.T.; Kandhare, A.D.; Zanwar, A.A.; Jagtap, S.D.; Katyare, S.S.; Bodhankar, S.L.; Hegde, M.V. Hepatoprotective effect of withanolide-rich fraction in acetaminophen-intoxicated rat: Decisive role of TNF-α, IL-1β, COX-II and iNOS. *Pharm. Biol.,* **2016**, *54*(11), 2394-2403.
[http://dx.doi.org/10.3109/13880209.2016.1157193] [PMID: 27043749]

[118] Kapil, A.; Koul, I.B.; Banerjee, S.K.; Gupta, B.D. Antihepatotoxic effects of major diterpenoid constituents of *Andrographis paniculata. Biochem. Pharmacol.,* **1993**, *46*(1), 182-185.
[http://dx.doi.org/10.1016/0006-2952(93)90364-3] [PMID: 8347130]

[119] Long, Y.; Lin, X.T.; Zeng, K.L.; Zhang, L. Efficacy of intramuscular matrine in the treatment of chronic hepatitis B. *Hepatobiliary Pancreat. Dis. Int.,* **2004**, *3*(1), 69-72.
[PMID: 14969841]

[120] Ikeda, K.; Arase, Y.; Kobayashi, M.; Saitoh, S.; Someya, T.; Hosaka, T.; Sezaki, H.; Akuta, N.; Suzuki, Y.; Suzuki, F.; Kumada, H. A long-term glycyrrhizin injection therapy reduces hepatocellular carcinogenesis rate in patients with interferon-resistant active chronic hepatitis C: A cohort study of 1249 patients. *Dig. Dis. Sci.,* **2006**, *51*(3), 603-609.
[http://dx.doi.org/10.1007/s10620-006-3177-0] [PMID: 16614974]

[121] Park, H.; Kim, Y.; Lee, E.; Lim, Y.; Kwon, O. Barley sprouts may have a hepatoprotective effect by reducing oxidative stress in habitual alcohol drinkers: A randomized, double-blind, placebo-controlled study. *Curr. Dev. Nutr.,* **2020**, *4*(2), nzaa052_039.
[http://dx.doi.org/10.1093/cdn/nzaa052_039]

[122] Panahi, Y.; Kianpour, P.; Mohtashami, R.; Atkin, S.L.; Butler, A.E.; Jafari, R.; Badeli, R.; Sahebkar, A. Efficacy of artichoke leaf extract in non-alcoholic fatty liver disease: A pilot double-blind randomized controlled trial. *Phytother. Res.,* **2018**, *32*(7), 1382-1387.
[http://dx.doi.org/10.1002/ptr.6073] [PMID: 29520889]

[123] Wah Kheong, C.; Nik Mustapha, N.R.; Mahadeva, S. A randomized trial of silymarin for the treatment of nonalcoholic steatohepatitis. *Clin. Gastroenterol. Hepatol.,* **2017**, *15*(12), 1940-1949.e8.
[http://dx.doi.org/10.1016/j.cgh.2017.04.016] [PMID: 28419855]

[124] Fried, MW; Navarro, VJ; Afhdal, N; Belle, SH; Wahad, AS; Hawke, RL Effect of silymarin (milk thistle) on liver disease in patients with chronic hepatitis C unsuccessfully treated with interferon therapy: A randomized controlled trial. *JAMA,* **2012**, *308*(3), 274-282.

[125] Chiu, H.F.; Fu, H.Y.; Lu, Y.Y.; Han, Y.C.; Shen, Y.C.; Venkatakrishnan, K.; Golovinskaia, O.; Wang, C.K. Triterpenoids and polysaccharide peptides-enriched *Ganoderma lucidum* : A randomized, double-blind placebo-controlled crossover study of its antioxidation and hepatoprotective efficacy in healthy volunteers. *Pharm. Biol.,* **2017**, *55*(1), 1041-1046.
[http://dx.doi.org/10.1080/13880209.2017.1288750] [PMID: 28183232]

[126] Chiou, Y.L.; Chyau, C.C.; Li, T.J.; Kuo, C.F.; Kang, Y.Y.; Chen, C.C.; Ko, W.S. Hepatoprotective effect of *Antrodia cinnamomea* Mycelium in patients with nonalcoholic steatohepatitis: A randomized, double-blind, placebo-controlled trial. *J. Am. Coll. Nutr.,* **2021**, *40*(4), 349-357.
[http://dx.doi.org/10.1080/07315724.2020.1779850] [PMID: 32657670]

CHAPTER 4

Hepatoprotective Role of Herbs and Herbal Formulations

Neetesh Kumar Jain[1,*] and **Nitu Singh**[2]

[1] *Department of Pharmacology, Modern Institute of Pharmaceutical Sciences, Indore, MP, India*

[2] *RGS College of Pharmacy, Itaunja, Lucknow, UP, India*

Abstract: The liver is an important organ in the body's metabolism and excretory system. The prevalence of many forms of hepatic illnesses is on the rise, resulting in a major increase in morbidity and mortality worldwide. Viral hepatitis, alcoholic/non-alcoholic fatty liver disease, liver fibrosis, cirrhosis, hepatocellular cancer, and drug-induced liver injury are all important health concerns that take millions of lives each year throughout the world. Pharmaceutical medications are frequently linked to liver injury, and so have limited efficacy in the treatment of liver diseases. As a result, herbal drugs have grown in popularity and are widely used. For a long time, herbal remedies have been utilized to treat liver problems. There are a variety of herbal preparations on the market. Herbal medicine has been used to treat liver disorders for thousands of years. A large range of medicinal plants have been examined as hepatoprotective agents in preclinical and clinical investigations. However, more thorough research is needed to screen and evaluate the usage of herbal medicines in the treatment of diverse liver illnesses. The goal of this review is to compile information on promising medicinal plants that have been tested in hepatotoxicity models using cutting-edge scientific methods. The damage to liver cells caused by various toxic chemicals (antibiotics, chemotherapeutic agents, carbon tetrachloride (CCl_4), thioacetamide (TAA), and microbes have been well studied. In this scenario, the current synthetic medications to treat liver problems promote more liver damage. The purpose of this chapter is to examine various hepatoprotective plants and herbal formulations.

Keywords: Carbon tetrachloride, Hepatoprotective agents, Hepatitis, Liver, Liver Disorders, Phytochemicals, Thioacetamide.

INTRODUCTION

The liver is a key organ that aids in the maintenance of the body's different physiological processes. It plays a major role in metabolism, secretion, and storage, among other bodily functions. It is involved in the detoxification and

* **Corresponding author Neetesh Kumar Jain:** Department of Pharmacology, Modern Institute of Pharmaceutical Sciences, Indore, India; Tel: 91-9479347077; E-mail: drnkjain9781@gmail.com

Sachin Kumar Jain, Ram Kumar Sahu, Priyanka Soni, Vishal Soni & Shiv Shankar Shukla (Eds.)

excretion of a variety of foreign and endogenous chemicals. Proteins, glycogen, different vitamins, and metals are all stored in it. It also plays a role in blood volume regulation by moving blood from the portal to the systemic circulation and its reticuloendothelial system, as well as contributing to the immune system [1]. The liver controls the majority of chemical levels in the blood and excretes bile. This aids in the removal of waste materials from the liver. The liver filters all of the blood that leaves the stomach and intestines. The liver processes blood, breaking down, balancing, and creating nutrients, as well as metabolizing medications into forms that are easier to use or harmless for the rest of the body. The liver cells, often known as hepatocytes, perform a variety of functions. The liver is responsible for more than 500 important activities (Fig. **1**). The following are some of the more well-known functions:

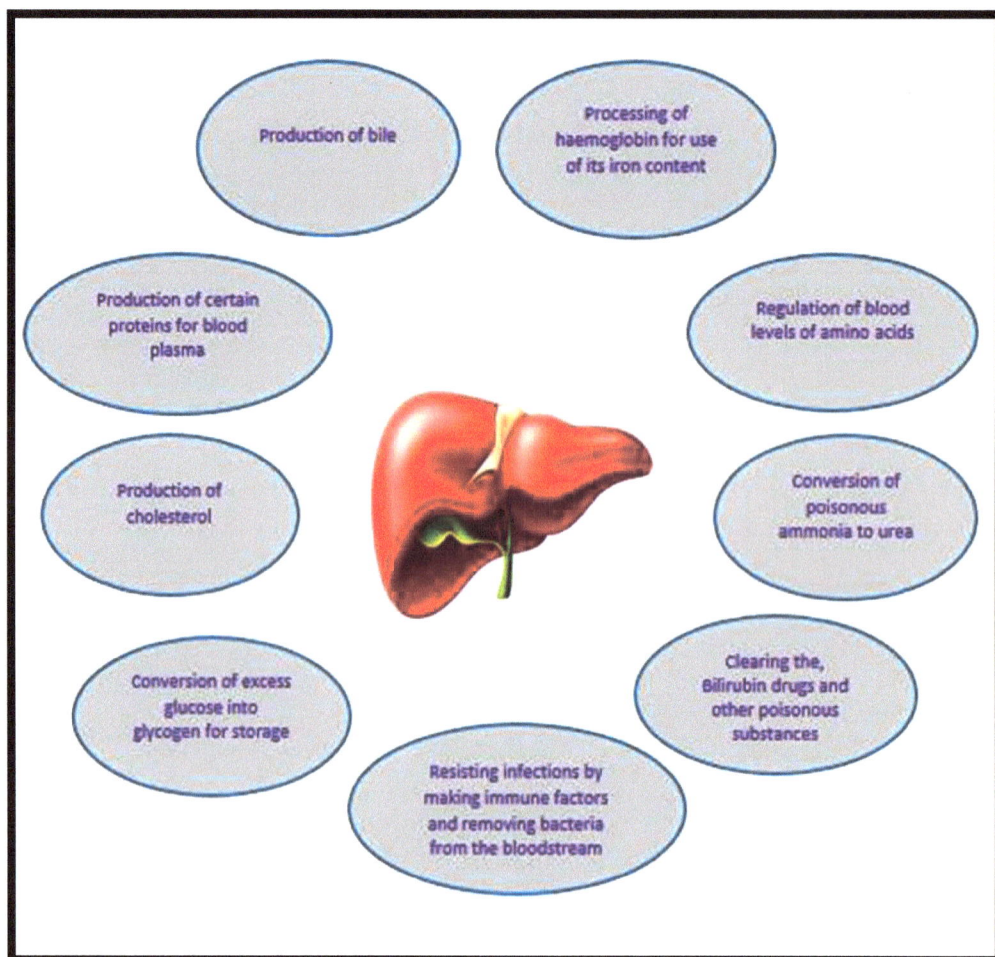

Fig. (1).   Functions of the liver [8].

- Bile production aids in the removal of waste and the breakdown of fats in the small intestine during digestion [2].
- The manufacture of specific proteins for blood plasma [3].
- Cholesterol and specific proteins are produced to aid in the transport of fats throughout the body.
- Storage of excess glucose as glycogen (which can subsequently be converted back into glucose for energy), as well as balancing and producing glucose when needed [4].
- Controlling the amounts of amino acids in the blood, which are the building blocks of proteins [5].
- Haemoglobin processing for the usage of iron content (the liver stores iron).
- Clearing the blood from drugs and other harmful compounds by converting toxic ammonia into urea (urea is a by-product of protein synthesis and is eliminated in the urine).
- Making immune factors and eliminating pathogens from the bloodstream to fight illnesses [6].
- Bilirubin clearance [7].

Because of its essential function in chemical clearance and modification, the liver is vulnerable to drug-induced damage [9]. The liver is vulnerable to a variety of disorders due to its strategic position and multifaceted functions. Any damage to it or impairment of its function has serious health consequences for the individual who is affected. Due to food choices, alcohol consumption, poor cleanliness, uncontrolled drug use, and smoking, liver problems are the most common health concern in underdeveloped countries. Liver diseases are a prominent source of mortality all over the world [10]. According to studies, liver problems cause between 18000 and 20000 death of people worldwide each year [11, 12]. About 2-5 percent of hospital admissions in the United States are related to liver injury, with 10% of them resulting in acute liver failure [13, 14]. Globally, the crude incidence of liver disease is 14 per 100000 people per year, while the standard incidence is 8.1 per 100000 people per year [15]. Acute liver failure affects up to 13% of people in wealthy countries like the United States but only 5% of people in tropical countries like India [16]. Non-inflammatory, inflammatory, and degenerative liver illnesses are all possible. Due to hepatic insufficiency, elevated levels of plasma total cholesterol, Low-density lipoprotein Cholesterol (LDL-C), and triacylglycerols (TGs) are linked to an increased risk of atherosclerosis and cardiovascular disease [17, 18]. Hepatotoxicity is caused by a variety of toxins, including carbon tetrachloride (CCl_4), thioacetamide, and acute or chronic alcohol intake, as well as diseases such as hepatitis A, B, and C, and medications, the latter of which is the most common culprit. Alcohol consumption causes the formation of free radicals, which leads to the development of hepatitis and cirrhosis [19]. Although viral infection is one of the leading causes of hepatic damage, over 18,000 people are known to die each year from liver cirrhosis induced by hepatitis. At this time, no artificial organ or technology can perform all of the activities of the liver. Liver dialysis, an experimental treatment for liver failure, can perform some activities. The liver is responsible for roughly 20% of total body oxygen use during rest.

Liver Diseases

Many liver illnesses are accompanied by jaundice, which is caused by elevated bilirubin levels in the body. Bilirubin is produced by the breakdown of haemoglobin in dead red blood cells, which is generally eliminated by the liver and expelled through the bile. Hepatitis, or liver inflammation, is caused by a variety of viruses, as well as toxic substances, autoimmune illnesses, and hereditary abnormalities. Cirrhosis of the liver is defined as the growth of fibrous tissue in the liver that kills hepatocytes. Viral hepatitis, alcohol intoxication, and other toxic chemicals can all induce liver cell death. Hemochromatosis is a genetic condition in which the body accumulates iron, causing long-term liver damage. Adenoma, "angioma," and focal nodular hyperplasia are benign tumors. Cancer of the liver as a primary tumor, cholangiocarcinoma, or cancer metastasis to other organs of the digestive system; Wilson disease is a hereditary condition in which the body accumulates copper. Bile is carried by primary sclerosing cholangitis, an inflammatory autoimmune illness. Primary biliary cirrhosis is an autoimmune illness that affects the small bile ducts. Budd-Chiari syndrome, also known as hepatic vein syndrome, is a condition that affects the liver. Gilbert's syndrome is a bilirubin metabolism condition caused by a genetic mutation. There are a variety of liver illnesses that affect children. Several specific clinical investigations that detect the presence or absence of usual enzymes, metabolites, or chemicals associated with regular activities can be used to verify proper liver function [20]. Despite significant breakthroughs in modern medicine, no fully effective medications exist to promote hepatic function, provide total organ protection, or aid in the regeneration of hepatic cells [21]. Furthermore, some medicines can cause negative or side effects. As a result, alternative medications for the treatment of hepatic illnesses must be identified, with the goal of making these drugs more effective and less harmful. The intake of certain fruits and the application of certain plants have played important roles in human health care. Traditional medicine, which is mostly based on plant materials, is used by around 80% of the world's population for health treatment [22, 23].

Role of Medicinal Plants in Hepatotoxicity

Plant materials have been employed in Ayurveda to protect the liver from various poisons and dietary factors. As a result, herbal medications have grown in popularity in recent years due to their safety and capacity to cure such disorders. These drugs are also incredibly cost-effective when used for a long time. Many medicinal plants found in various parts of India have been identified as hepatoprotective medications and are widely utilized to treat liver diseases. Hepatoprotective action can be found in a variety of plants and polyherbal preparations. Hepatoprotective action has been claimed for around 160 phytochemicals [24]. Over 87 plants are used in India, with 33 of them being patented and having exclusive multi-ingredient plant compositions [25]. We reviewed some common herbal plants with hepatoprotective properties to underline the relevance of their use.

Aegle Marmelos

The most effective treatment for doxorubicin-induced hepatotoxicity is *Aegle marmelos* (Fig. **2A**) leaves extract at a dose of 25 mg/kg [26]. In a study with diabetic rats induced with streptozotocin, it was discovered that the changes in hepatic parameters, such as liver fibrosis, vein dilatation, hepatocyte organization, depletion of distinctive concentric, and reduction of glycogen content, had returned to normal levels [27]. *A. marmelos* fruit pulp is investigated for CCl_4 - induced hepatoprotective activity in pre and post-treatment procedures [28]. Liver damage markers such as Serum Glutamic-oxalacetic transaminase (SGOT), Serum glutamate pyruvate transaminase (SGPT), alkaline phosphatase (ALP), and bilirubin are decreased by a good amount in CCl_4 -only groups. Post-treatment scores well than the pre-treatment schedule. The reverse result is found for *A. marmelos* seed experimented in the same way [29]. Eugenol extracted from *A. marmelos* leaf has been found to exhibit hepatoprotective activity [30]. The hepatoprotective effect of *A. marmelos* has been further confirmed by the investigation where they have found rutin present in bael, possibly the reason behind the said activity. Here the increased Tumour Necrosis Factor-alpha (TNF-α) level has decreased, also the efficacy is similar to the action of silymarin. Piperine, in combination with bael extract, has shown effective outcomes against CCl_4 administered liver problems [31].

Andrographis Paniculata

The leaf extract and andrographolide were evaluated against carbon tetrachloride CCl_4 induced hepatic microsomal lipid peroxidation in comparative research. Only the leaf extract, not the andrographolide, totally prevented microsomal lipid peroxidation in vitro caused by high concentrations of CCl_4, indicating that the hepatoprotective action is not entirely attributable to the presence of andrographolide [32]. Rana and Avadhoot [33] showed similar efficacy of crude alcohol extracts of *Andrographis paniculata* leaves (Fig. **2B**) against CCl4-

induced liver injury. Handa and Sharma [34] found that against CCl_4-induced liver injury, andrographolide, methanol extract of the entire plant, and andrographolide-free methanol extract improved liver histology in rats by 48.6%, 32%, and 15%, respectively. After CCl4-induced liver injury, Verma *et al.* [35] investigated the efficacy of an ethanolic extract of *Andrographis paniculata* to restore several enzymes. Along with various extracts of *Andrographis paniculata*, phytoconstituents such as andrographolide, neoandrographolide,14-dexoyandrographolide, and14-deoxy-11,12-didehydroandrographolide have been shown to exhibit hepatoprotective properties [36, 37].

Allium Sativum

Allium sativum (Fig. **2C**) demonstrated a hepatoprotective effect in Wistar rats when it came to anti-tubercular drug-induced hepatotoxicity. In this experiment, the medicine Isoniazid (INH) was discovered to have a hepatotoxic effect. The values of Serum alanine transaminase (ALT), Serum aspartate transaminase (AST), Serum Alkaline phosphatase (ALP), and total bilirubin in the blood were all abnormally high. Hepatotoxicity is indicated by elevated levels of these biochemical markers in the serum. Garlic and silymarin had a hepatoprotective effect in model animals when given at a level of 0.25 g/kg per day. In this study, garlic was found to be beneficial in reducing INH-induced hepatotoxicity [38]. Garlic extracts were found to have a hepatoprotective effect on Cadmium (Cd)-induced oxidative damage in rats. The hepatic activities of ALT, AST, and alkaline phosphatase were reduced by *Allium sativum* extract, whereas the plasma activities of ALT and AST were elevated. Cd-induced oxidative damage in the rat liver is reduced by a moderate dosage of *Allium sativum* extracts, most likely due to lower Hepatic lipid peroxidation (LPO) and an improved antioxidant defense mechanism that could not prevent and protect against Cd-induced hepatotoxicity [39]. Chemical substances from *Allium sativum* have been shown to reduce iron liver excess [40]. The hepatoprotective benefits of *Allium sativum*, ginger (*Zingiber officinale*), and vitamin E against CCl_4-induced liver damage in male Wistar albino rats were investigated in another investigation. In rats pretreated with garlic, ginger, vitamin E, and various combinations of garlic and ginger, serum alanine aminotransferase, aspartate aminotransferase, and alkaline phosphatase levels reduced considerably 24 hours after CCl_4 treatment compared to rats treated with simply CCl_4. LPO expressed by serum malondialdehyde (MDA) was assayed to assess the severity of liver damage by CCl_4, including the extent of hepatoprotection by garlic, ginger, and vitamin E. MDA concentration was significantly decreased in rats pretreated with garlic, ginger, vitamin E, and various mixtures of garlic and ginger compared to the rats administered by CC14 alone. In rats treated with CCl_4 alone, histological analysis of the liver revealed substantial infiltration of inflammatory cells, even though the change in the normal architecture of the hepatic cells was significantly reduced in pre-treated rats [41]. The hepatoprotective efficacy of *Allium sativum* extract at a dose of 300 mg/kg body weight, given intraperitoneally for 14 days before the induction of D-galactosamine(DGalN) and lipopolysaccharide (LPS), was, against DGalN/LPS-induced hepatitis in rats. The altered parameters (ALT, AST, ALP, lactate dehydrogenase (LDH), gamma-glutamyl transferase, bilirubin, LPO, tumor necrosis factor, and myeloperoxidase activity level, total cholesterol, triglycerides, free fatty acids, and antioxidant enzyme activities) were helped to reach nearly normal control values after pretreatment with aqueous *Allium sativum* extract. Aqueous *Allium sativum* extract could afford significant protection in the DGalN/LPS-induced hepatic damage easing [42]. The synergistic effect of *A. sativum* extract and silymarin on N-nitrosodiethylamine and CCl$_4$-induced hepatotoxicity in male albino rats was discovered [43].

Allium Cepa

It has been used for centuries to treat intestinal infections, ear aches, eye infections, headaches, sleepiness, urinary tract infections, burning ulcers, and cough [44]. It is also used for its antiviral, antifungal, antibacterial, and anti-parasitic properties, as well as antihypertensive, hypoglycemic, antithrombotic, antihyperlipidemic, anti-inflammatory, and antioxidant properties [45 - 47]. *Allium cepa* (Fig. **2D**) possesses hepatoprotective properties against paracetamol-induced liver injury in rats, according to Ozougwu and Eyo [48]. In adult male albino Wistar rats, aqueous bulb extract of *A. cepa* has hepatoprotective properties against hepatotoxicity [49]. Ige *et al.* [50] discovered that *Allium cepa* could protect rats from cadmium-induced hepatotoxicity. Lee *et al* [51]. also discovered that *Allium cepa* extract could rescue mice from acetaminophen-induced liver injury.

Azadirachta Indica

Bitter active components can be found in several parts of the plant (Fig. **2E**) [52]. It reduced blood glucose levels and slowed the progression of stomach ulcers [53]. The hepatoprotective efficacy of aqueous, alcoholic, ethyl acetate and petroleum ether extracts of *A. indica* leaves was observed by Patel *et al.* [54]. Fresh juice of young stem bark of *A. indica* was also tested for antioxidant and hepatoprotective activities against CCl4-induced liver damage [55]. The findings suggested that the antioxidant and hepatoprotective properties of fresh neem juice may be linked to its free radical scavenging activity. In rats, Chattopadhyay *et al.* [56] found that *A. indica* leaves had a hepatoprotective effect against paracetamol-induced liver damage.

Berberis Vulgaris

The effects of hydroalcoholic extract of *Berberis vulgaris* (Fig. **2F**) leaves on hepatic protection were assessed in rats against carbon tetrachloride-induced hepatotoxicity. The *B. vulgaris* extract in every three doses (40, 80, and 120 mg/kg) of weight caused a significant decrease in hepatic enzymes level [57]. In another study, the preventive effect of *Berberis vulgaris* L. extract against CCl_4-induced acute hepatotoxicity in mouse liver as well as the effects of β-cyclodextrin complexation in hepatoprotective therapeutic formulations, is evaluated. Internucleosomal DNA fragmentation induced by CCl_4 was reduced in the group which received the non-formulated extract and was absent in the group which received the formulated extract. Taken together, results suggested that *Berberis vulgaris*/β-cyclodextrin treatment prevents hepatic injury induced by CCl_4 [58]. Intraperitoneal injection of berberine in rats at a dose of 0.5–5 mg/kg, on the other hand, reduced the oxidative stress caused by tert-butyl hydroperoxide toxicity [59]. There have been a few investigations on the oral treatment of rats with *Berberis vulgaris* root extract. The effective dose for protecting the liver was 900 mg/kg, which is 30 times greater than the usual dose utilized in several traditional medical systems [60].

Boerhavia Diffusa

Due to their safety and efficacy, the roots of *Boerhavia diffusa* (Punarnava) (Fig. **2G**) are used to treat a variety of liver ailments. Punarnava is a Sanskrit term that means "one who renews the body." Punarnava has long been regarded as an important medicinal herb in India. In India, South America, and Africa, *B. diffusa* (family Nyctaginaceae) is an essential medicinal herb for treating liver problems [61]. *B. diffusa* is useful in treating hepatotoxicity induced by paracetamol and acetaminophen [62 - 65]. Punarnava is also important for the treatment of jaundice [66, 67]. Shameela *et al.* found that giving *B. diffusa* at 150 mg/kg body weight/day for 45 days cures hepatitis caused by isoproterenol in rats. *B. diffusa's* hepatoprotective benefits could be attributed to its oxidant properties, membrane-stabilizing action, or ability to maintain near-normal levels of free radical enzymes and glutathione (GSH), which protect the hepatic membrane from oxidative damage by lowering lipid protection [68].

Cassia Fistula

Inducing hepatotoxicity in rats with paracetamol revealed hepatoprotective action of the n-heptane extract of *Cassia fistula* (Fabaceae) leaves (Fig. **2H**). At a dose of 400 mg/kg body weight, the treatment extract was administered. It showed a strong protective impact by reducing serum Glutamic-oxalacetic transaminase (SGOT) and glutamic-pyruvic transaminase (SGPT), bilirubin, and alkaline phosphatase levels when taken orally. The effects produced were comparable to that of a standard hepatoprotective agent [69]. The protective effects of Cassia seed ethanol extract are reported against carbon tetrachloride-induced liver injury in mice [70]. The protective effect of *Cassia fistula* Linn. on diethyl nitrosamine-induced hepatocellular damage and oxidative stress is reported in ethanol-pretreated rats [71]. The protective effect of *Cassia fistula* fruit extract against bromobenzene-induced liver injury in mice is also reported [72].

Cissus Quadrangularis

At a dose of 500mg/kg of BW p.o., the methanolic extract of *Cissus quadrangularis* showed hepatoprotective efficacy against isoniazid-produced hepatotoxicity in rats. *Cissus quadrangularis* (Fig. **2I**) have protective effects by reducing increased levels of aspartate transaminase, alanine transaminase, alkaline phosphatase, and bilirubin. The presence of phytochemical ingredients and antioxidant properties are responsible for *Cissus quadrangularis* hepatoprotective action [73]. Swamy *et al.* [74] investigated the hepatoprotective activity of the methanolic extract of *C. quadrangularis* against rifampicin-induced hepatotoxicity in rats. It was concluded that the mechanism of hepatoprotection might be attributed to its antioxidant activity, especially the presence of β–carotene. The plant affords hepatoprotection through its antioxidant and insulin-sensitizing activities [75]. It also showed anti-lipid peroxidative, free-radical scavenging properties and ameliorated liver damage through an increase in antioxidant enzyme activities [76].

Curcuma Longa

In jaundice, rhizome powder combined with amla juice is utilized [77]. Curcumin is the most frequent antioxidant ingredient of *Curcuma longa* rhizome (Fig. **2J**) extract. It has been shown to increase apoptosis in injured hepatocytes, suggesting that curcumin may protect the liver by reducing inflammatory effects and fibrogenesis [78]. When given orally in doses of 250 mg/kg and 500 mg/kg, the ethanolic extract of *Curcuma Longa* rhizomes showed a significant hepatoprotective effect, with the protective effect being dose-dependent [79]

Eclipta Alba

Eclipta alba (Fig. **2K**) has hepatoprotective properties. Tabassum and Agrawal investigated the effects of *E.alba* on paracetamol-induced hepatocellular damage in mice [80]. The levels of serum alanine aminotransferase were substantially greater in animals given paracetamol and significantly lower in those given *E. alba*. The levels recovered to normal in the group of mice given 250 mg/100 g *E. alba* and paracetamol. The hepatoprotective activity of *E. alba* was investigated by Saxena *et al.* by analyzing biochemical parameters such as superoxide dismutase, glutathione reductase, lipid peroxide, catalase, glutathione peroxide, ascorbic acid, and -tocopherol. In the rat liver, the ethyl acetate fraction *of E. alba* enhances both enzymatic and nonenzymatic antioxidant status [81]. Methanolic extract and subfractions of leaves and chloroform extract and subfractions of roots of *E. alba* have a hepatoprotective effect. In Wistar albino rats, carbon tetrachloride-induced liver damage and lysosomal enzyme levels were studied. The methanolic and chloroform extracts of *E. alba* leaves and roots exhibited substantial activity, causing a 73 percent and 48 percent decrease in lysosomal enzyme, respectively [82].

Ginseng Species

The dried root of Panax spp. (Fig. **2L**) (family Araliaceae), such as *Panax ginseng* Meyer (PG, Asian Ginseng or Korean Ginseng), *Panax quiquifolius* L. (PQ, American Ginseng), and *Panax notoginseng* PN (Burk.) [83, 84], is known as ginseng. Ginsengs (PG, PQ, and PN) and their constituents have been proven to be effective in treating a variety of liver ailments. Red Ginseng (RG) extract enhances liver function by reducing steatosis and oxidative stress caused by ethanol [85]. Elevations in serum aspartate transaminase (AST) and alanine transaminase (ALT) are associated with chronic ethanol-induced liver damage. After short-term ethanol administration, however, pretreatment with RG extract kept serum ALT activity and malondialdehyde (MDA) concentrations below normal limits [86]. *Panax Notoginseng* reduces serum AST and ALT elevations caused by persistent ethanol-induced hepatotoxicity [87]. In rats with ethanol-induced liver damage, *Panax Notoginseng* decreases liver ALT and AST levels, collagen fibers deposition, and transforming growth factor (TGF)-1 expression, all of which are associated with an increase in the expression amount of SMA/MAD homologous protein 7 (Smad7) [88]. Cirrhosis of the liver, which precedes hepatic cancer, necessitates constant monitoring. By lowering hepatitis virus titers, RG and its constituents, ginsenosides Rg1 and Rb1 have been demonstrated to have a hepatoprotective impact against hepatitis virus A [89].

Hemidesmus Indicus

The methanolic root extract of *Hemidesmus indicus* (500 mg/kg, p.o.) showed hepatoprotective activity against paracetamol and carbon tetrachloride-induced hepatotoxicity in rats [90, 91]. Rifampicin and Isoniazid (INH) caused liver damage and were protected by an ethanolic extract of *Hemidesmus indicus* roots. Isocitrate dehydrogenase, ketoglutarate dehydrogenase, succinate dehydrogenase, malate dehydrogenase, cytochrome C oxidase, and NADH dehydrogenase activities were not affected by extract (100mg/kg b.w./day for 15 days). These effects are most likely due to coumarinolignoids, such as coumarin. Hemidesmin-I and hemidesmin-II, both of which have free radical scavenging activity [92], as well as a 50 percent aqueous ethanolic extract of *Hemidesmus indicus* (400 mg/kg, daily orally), demonstrated similar hepatoprotective effects against carbon tetrachloride (CCl_4)-induced liver damage. Methanolic extract of *Hemidesmus indicus* roots (Fig. **2M**) showed hepatoprotective benefits against carbon tetrachloride (CCl_4) and paracetamol-caused liver injury. These effects were related to its free radical scavenging and anti-lipid peroxidative activities [93]. In rats with hepatic damage, the extract reduced elevated levels of serum glutamate pyruvate transaminase (SGPT), serum glutamate oxaloacetate transaminase (SGOT), alkaline phosphatase (ALP), total and direct bilirubin [94]. The ethanolic extract of *Hemidesmus indicus* also protected against ethanol-induced liver injury. The extract dramatically reduced liver collagen and hydroxyproline concentration, lipid peroxidation, and increased liver collagen solubility and ascorbic acid levels. The extract also reduced the activities of matrix metalloproteinase-2 and matrix metalloproteinase-9, which are involved in the destruction of extracellular matrix during ethanol intoxication [95, 96].

Ocimum Sanctum

In a study of the hepatoprotective effect of *Ocimum sanctum* (Fig. **2N**) alcoholic leaves extract against paracetamol-induced liver damage in albino rats, Lahon *et al.* found that *Ocimum sanctum* alcoholic leaf extract demonstrated considerable hepatoprotective action and synergism with silymarin. The Ayurvedic medication *O. sanctum* is used to cure a common cold, headaches, stomach issues, inflammation, heart illness, poisoning, and malaria [97]. This plant has been stated to have anabolic, hypotensive, cardiac depressive, smooth muscle relaxant, anti-fertility, and anti-stress properties by several studies [98]. Several researchers have proved that *O. sanctum* has hepatoprotective capability against paracetamol, CCl4, and lead-induced liver injury [99, 100].

Phyllanthus Emblica

The ability of the medicinal plant *Phyllanthus emblica* (Fig. **2O**) to protect rats from paracetamol-induced hepatotoxicity was investigated using histological analysis of liver cells. The animals were given *Phyllanthus emblica* aqueous extracts of 100 and 200 mg/kg/day, p.o., for 14 days. The total blood cell count in each animal group was also calculated. *Phyllanthus emblica* (100-200mg/kg) improved the cell viability of rat hepatocytes treated with paracetamol. The hepatotoxicity of rats pre-treated with *Phyllanthus emblica* at oral dosages of 100-200 mg/kg 4 hours before paracetamol administration was reduced. The hepatoprotective effect of *Phyllanthus emblica* was demonstrated in a study using an aqueous extract of the medicinal plant's fruits [101]. In rat studies, alcoholic and aqueous extracts of Emblica fruits showed hepatoprotective effects. Hepatic insults include tuberculosis medicines, arsenic, ethanol, thioacetamide, carbon tetrachloride, and cyclophosphamide. The trials revealed protective and restorative histological and/or enzymatic effects. Hepatic fibrosis severity was reduced, while renal and pancreatic indices were improved in several studies [102 - 112].

Picrorhiza Kurroa

Picrorhiza kurroa roots (Fig. **2U**) have been found to have a hepatoprotective effect in a variety of liver injury models. The crude extract and extracted active principles of the roots have been demonstrated to protect the liver from various forms of drug-induced injuries. *P. kurroa* isolated compounds have also been shown to exhibit hepatoprotective potential. Using hydro-alcoholic extracts of *Picrorhiza kurroa*, rats with non-alcoholic fatty liver disease (NAFLD) were healed. At a dose of 400mg/kg, it significantly lowered the lipid content of the liver [113]. In vitro, Kutkin from *Picrorhiza kurroa* showed considerable curative action against thioacetamide, galactosamine, and carbon tetrachloride toxicity in primary cultured rat hepatocytes [114]. The liver injury was generated in 16 mice by injecting carbon tetrachloride (CCl_4) thrice a week for nine weeks. Ten days before the CCl_4 injection, eight of them were given daily feedings of *Picrorhiza kurroa* extract (12 mg/Kg). Olive oil was administered to control mice (n = 6) for the same time. The histology of liver tissues and serum indicators of liver damage were investigated. Total thiol, hepatic glutathione, glucose 6-phosphate dehydrogenase, catalase, lipid peroxidation, and plasma membrane-bound Na+/K+ ATPase were also measured. *Picrorhiza kurroa* extract provides considerable protection against CCl_4-induced liver damage [115]. Picrorhiza's active ingredient was studied in another investigation. Picrorhiza kurroa had a dose-dependent hepatoprotective effect against oxytetracycline-induced liver damage in rats. *Picrorhiza kurroa* root powder 375 mg three times a day for two weeks and matching placebo were provided in a randomized, double-blind, placebo-controlled experiment to individuals diagnosed with acute viral hepatitis. Between the placebo and *Picrorhiza kurroa* groups, there was a significant difference in bilirubin, SGOT, and SGPT values [116].

Silybum Marianum

Silymarin (Fig. **2P**) has been used as a natural medicine to treat liver disorders in rural areas [117]. In most liver illnesses, such as cirrhosis, hepatitis, and jaundice, silymarin protects and enhances liver cell regeneration [118]. Silymarin has anti-oxidant, anti-lipid peroxidant, anti-fibrotic, and immune-modulatory activities, and it aids liver regeneration [119, 120]. The capacity of silymarin to block free radicals formed by the metabolism of harmful chemicals such as ethanol, acetaminophen, and carbon tetrachloride is responsible for its hepatoprotective and antioxidant properties. Free radicals have been shown to harm cellular membranes and produce lipoperoxidation. Silymarin raises hepatic glutathione levels, which may help the liver's antioxidant defenses. Silymarin has also been demonstrated to stimulate RNA polymerase I activity, which boosts protein synthesis in hepatocytes. In a preliminary human trial, Silymarin treatment resulted in a modest increase in the survival of cirrhotic alcoholism patients compared to untreated controls [121, 122].

Solanum Nigrum

In rats, the protective properties of *Solanum nigrum* (Fig. **2Q**) aqueous extract against liver damage was tested using carbon tetrachloride (CCl_4)-induced chronic hepatotoxicity. The findings of this study suggest that *Solanum nigrum* can protect rats' livers from CCl_4-induced oxidative damage, and this hepatoprotective effect may be due to its modulation of detoxification enzymes, as well as its antioxidant and free radical scavenging properties [123]. Other studies have shown that oral administration of *Solanum nigrum* inhibits thioacetamide-induced hepatic fibrosis in mice, most likely through lowering TGF-1 production [124].

Terminalia Arjuna

The hepatoprotective activity of an aqueous extract of *Terminalia arjuna* bark (Fig. **2R**) against Isoniazid-induced acute liver injury in albino rats was examined. When albino rats were given Isoniazid (100mg/kg), blood levels of biochemical indicators such as SGPT, SGOT, ALP, Acyl carrier protein (ACP), Bilirubin, and Protein were dramatically raised, whereas antioxidant enzymes GSH and Superoxide dismutase (SOD) were depleted. This showed that a 200mg/kg dose of aqueous extract of *Terminalia arjuna* bark effectively lowered high levels of biochemical markers. SOD and GSH levels were also raised by the extract. These findings suggested that *Terminalia arjuna* aqueous extract could be useful in the treatment of Isoniazid-induced hepatic damage and various liver disorders [125]. The protecting role of the aqueous extract of the bark of T. arjuna (TA; 50 mg kg-1 b.wt.) on CCl4 (1 mL kg-1 b.wt.) induced oxidative stress, and resultant dysfunction in the livers and kidneys of mice was examined. Results showed that CCl_4 caused a marked increase in serum levels of GPT and ALP. Thiobarbituric acid reactive substances (TBARS) levels also rise significantly whereas GSH, SOD, oxidative stress catalase (CAT), and glutathione-S-transferase (GST) levels were decreased in the liver and kidney tissue homogenates of CCl_4 treated mice. Aqueous extract of TA successfully prevented the alterations of these effects in the experimental animals. The aqueous extract of the bark of *Terminalia arjuna* could protect the liver and kidney tissues against CCl_4-induced oxidative stress, probably by increasing antioxidative defense activity [126].

Tinospora Cordifolia

The effects of various *Tinospora cordifolia* (Fig. **2S**) extracts on carbon tetrachloride (CCl_4)-induced liver damage in rats were examined. Wistar albino rats were given 200mg/kg body weight of petroleum ether, ethanol, and aqueous extracts of various sections of the plant, including the leaf, stem, and root. The results showed that the extract supplied greatly reduced the toxic effects of CCl_4 and aided in hepatocyte regeneration. According to these findings, *T. Cordifolia* leaf extracts are effective hepatoprotective against carbon tetrachloride-induced hepatotoxicity [127].

Trigonella-foenum-graecum

Trigonella leaf is high in calcium, iron, beta-carotene, and other phytonutrients. Culinary uses include leaves and seeds [128 - 130]. Flavonoids, polysaccharides, saponins, fibers, and alkaloids such as trigocoumarin, choline, and trigonelline are the primary chemical ingredients of *Trigonella* [131]. *Trigonella* leaf extracts have been shown to have cytoprotective, antioxidant, and hepatoprotective activities by Singh *et al.* [132], suggesting that they could be employed as dietary supplements or in liver disease formulations. Tripathi and Chandra [133] found that Trigonella's antioxidative capacity protects liver tissue from deltamethrin (DM)-induced toxicity. Increased levels of LPO and GSH and reduced antioxidant activity such as SOD, GST, and catalase indicate that DM causes oxidative stress in the rat liver. The *Trigonella* exposure resulted in a considerable recovery in these parameters' changed levels. On the basis of the foregoing, it is possible to conclude that Trigonella has antioxidative and antilipidemic properties. It can also help with hepatotoxicity caused by pesticides. The extract was prepared from dried seeds of Trigonella (Fig. **2T**) that have shown hepatoprotective activity in a rat model of thioacetamide-induced liver cirrhosis [134]. *Trigonella* methanol extract has a potent hepatoprotective action against CCl_4-induced toxicity [135].

Table 1. Herbs used as Hepatoprotective agents

S. No	Botanical Name	Family	Part Used	Ref. No
1.	*Aegle marmelos*	Rutaceae	Leaves, Fruit pulp and seeds	[26, 28, 29]
2	*Andrographis paniculata*	Acanthaceae	Leaves and Whole plant	[32, 34]
3	*Allium sativum*	Liliaceae	Bulb	[38 - 43]

(Table 1) cont.....

S. No	Botanical Name	Family	Part Used	Ref. No
4	*Allium Cepa*	Liliaceae	Bulb	[44 - 51]
5	*Azadirachta indica*	Meliaceae	Leaves, Barks	[54, 55]
6	*Berberis vulgaris*	Berberidaceae	Leaves, Root, Bark	[57 - 60]
7	*Boerhavia diffusa*	Nyctaginaceae	Leaves and Root	[61 - 68]
8	*Cassia fistula*	Fabaceae	Leaves, seeds, fruits	[69 - 72]
9	*Cissus quadrangularis*	Vitaceae	Stem	[73 - 75]
10	*Curcuma longa*	Zingiberaceae	Root tuber	[77 - 79]
11	*Eclipta alba*	Asteraceae	Leaves and Roots	[80 - 82]
12	*Panax ginseng*	Araliaceae	Root	[83 - 89]
13	*Hemidesmus indicus*	Apocynaceae	Root	[91 - 95]
14	*Ocimum sanctum*	Lamiaceae	Leaves	[96 - 100]
15	*Phyllanthus emblica*	Euphorbiaceae	Fruit	[101 - 112]
16	*Picrorhiza kurroa*	Plantaginaceae	Roots	[113 - 116]
17	*Silybum marianum* L	Asteraceae	Seeds	[117]
18	*Solanum nigrum*	Solanaceae	Fruits	[117, 118]
19	*Terminalia arjuna*	Combretaceae	Bark	[119, 120]
20	*Tinospora cordifolia*	Menispermaceae	Leaves, Root, Stem	[121]
21	*Trigonella-foenum-graecum*	Fabaceae	Leaves and Seeds	[122 - 129]

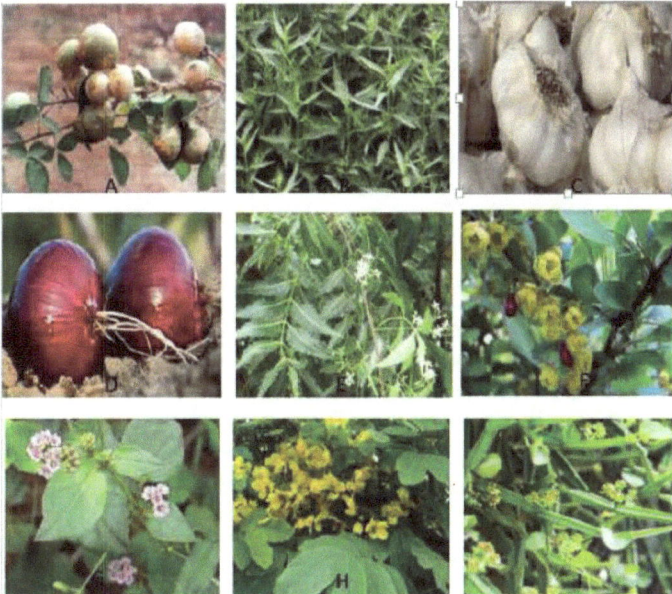

(Fig. 2) contd.....

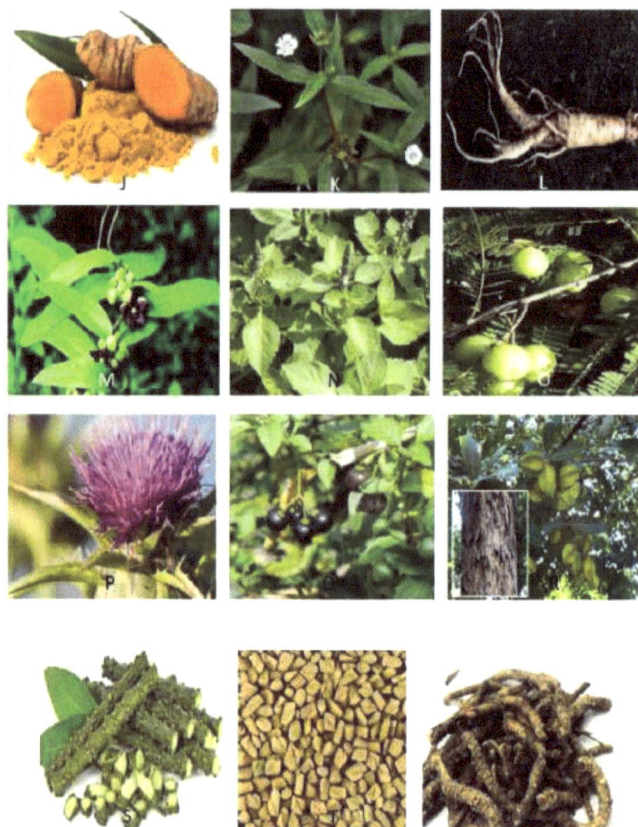

Fig. (2). (A) Leaves and fruits of Aegle marmelos (B) Leaves of Andrographis paniculata (C) Bulb of Allium sativum (D) Bulbs of Allium cepa (E). Leaves and Flowers of Azadirachta indica (F) Leaves, Fruits, and flowers of Berberis vulgaris (G) Flower and leaves of Boerhavia diffusa (H) Leaves and flowers of Cassia fistula (I) Leaves and flowers of Cissus quadrangularis [136 - 144]. Rhizome of Curcuma Longa (K). Flowers and leaves of Eclipta alba (L) Roots of Ginseng (M) Flower and leaves of Hemidesmus indicus . (N) Flower and leaves of Ocimum sanctum (O) Fruits and leaves of Phyllanthus emblica (P) Flower of Silybum marianum (Q) Fruits and Leaves of Solanum nigrum. (R) Bark, Fruits and Leaves of Terminalia arjuna [145 - 153]. (S)Stem of Tinospora cordifolia (T) Seeds of Trigonella-foenum-graecum (U) Roots Picrorhiza kurroa [154 - 156].

Hepatoprotective Polyherbal Formulations

Tinospora species are used to make Guduchi Satwa, an Ayurvedic medication. It has been used to treat liver problems since ancient times. Tejaswi Chavan *et al.* tested the hepatoprotective properties of Satwa made from three different types of Tinospora (*Tinospora cordifolia, Tinospora sinensis,* and Neem-Guduchi) against alcohol-induced hepatotoxicity (Table **2**). In the rats treated with *T. sinensis* Satwa, improvements in hepatic function, stabilization of serum and liver lipid profiles, and increased levels of antioxidant enzymes and oxidative-stress indicators were found. Neem-Guduchi Satwa was discovered to have a specific activity in lipid profile maintenance [157].

Table 2. Hepatoprotective formulations with their constituents

S. No	Name of Formulation	Constituents	References
1	Satwa	*Tinospora cordifolia, Tinospora sinensis,* and Neem-Guduchi	157
2	Punarnavashtak kwath	*Boerhaavia diffusa* Linn., *Picrorhiza kurroa* Royle ex Benth. *Tinospora cordifolia* (Willd.) Miers), *Zingiber officinalis* Rosc., *Berberis aristata* DC, *Terminalia chebula* Retz, *Azadirachta indica* A. Juss. and *Tricosanthes dioica* Roxb.	158
3.	Rohitakarista	*Aphanamixis polystachya* (Wall.) Parker, *Woodfordia fruticosa* (Linn.) Kurz. *Piper longum* Linn. (Root), *Piper longum* Linn. (Seed), *Zingiber officinale* Rosc., *Cinnamomum tamala* Ness, *Cinnamomum zeylanicum*Bl., *Elettaria cardamomum* (Linn.) Maton., *Phyllanthus emblica* Linn., *Terminalia chebula* (Gaertn.) Retz., *Terminalia belerica*Roxb	166
4	Livshis	*Aloe barbadensis* Mill., *Andrographis paniculata* Wall. ex Nees., *Asteracantha longifolia* Nees., *Berberis chitria* Lindl., *Fumaria parviflora* Lam., *Phyllanthus fraternus* Webs., *Picrorhiza kurroa* Royle ex Benth., *Phyllanthus fraternus* Webs.,	170
5	Livergen	*Andrographis paniculata, Apium graveolens, Berberis lycium, Carum copticum, Cichorium intybus, Cyperus rotundus, Eclipta alba, Ipomoea turpethum, Oldenlandia corymbosa, Picrorhiza kurroa, Plumbago zeylanica, Trigonella foenum graecum, Solanum nigrum, Tephrosia purpurea, Terminalia arjuna,* and *Terminalia chebula.*	171
6	Himoliv	*Phyllanthus niruri, Eclipta alba, Fumaria indica, Boerhavia diffusa, Ocimum sanctum,Rosa centifolia, Plumbago zeylanica, Berberis aristata, Tinospora cordifolia, Hemidesmus indicus, Rheum emodi, Cichorium intybus, Terminalia chebula, Andrographis paniculata, Tecomella undulate* and *Picrorhiza kurroa*	172
7	Hepax	*Plumbago zeylanica, Picrorrhiza kurroa, Piper nigrum, Zingiber officinale, Sodii carbonas impura, Phyllanthus emblica, Terminalia chebula, Calcii oxidum* and *Potassii carbonas impura*	173
8	BV-7310	*Phyllanthus niruri, Tephrosia purpurea, Boerhavia diffusa,* and *Andrographis paniculata*	175
9	Normeta®	Ashwagandha (*Withania somnifera*, Guduchi (*Tinospora cordifolia*), Gokshura (*Tribulus terrestris*), Amalaki (*Emblica officinalis*), Shatavari (*Asparagus racemosus*), Sunthi (*Zingiber officinale*) Pimpali (*Piper longum*), Mariach (*Piper nigrum*) Yasthimadhu (*Glycyrrhiza glabra*) Kapikachhu (*Mucuna pruriens*) Vridhdaruk (*Argyreia speciosa*) Draksha (*Vitis vinifera*), Tvak (*Cinnamomum zeylanicum*) Lavang (*Eugenia caryophyllus*)*Syzygium aromaticum*)	177

Punarnavashtak kwath (PNK) is an Ayurvedic polyherbal mixture (Table **2**) used to treat hepatic problems and asthma, according to the Ayurvedic literature Bhaishajya Ratnavali [158]. In rats, an aqueous extract of *B. diffusa* thinner roots showed a hepatoprotective effect in vivo [64]. The active components of *P. kurroa* were found to be helpful in reducing liver damage caused by a variety of hazardous substances [159]. In CCl_4-induced hepatopathy in goats, *T. cordifolia* showed considerable in vivo hepatoprotective action and in vitro inactivating capability against Hepatitis B and E surface antigens [160]. Because of its direct radical scavenging capacity, the aqueous ethanol extract of *Z. officinalis* displayed hepatoprotective effects against acetaminophen-induced acute toxicity [161]. Both paracetamol and CCl4-induced liver damage were shown to be protected by *B. aristata* and berberine (an alkaloid from *B. aristata*) [162]. The hepatotoxicity caused by the administration of rifampicin, isoniazid, and pyrazinamide was reported to be prevented by *T. chebula* extract [163]. In ferrous sulfate ($FeSO_4$)-intoxicated rats, *T. dioica* was found to be a hepatoprotective agent [164]. PNK's hepatoprotective efficacy was examined by Vaishali N. Shah *et al.* in order to support its traditional use. PNK administration resulted in strong hepatoprotective effects, as seen by lower levels of blood liver marker enzymes such as aspartate transaminase, serum alanine transaminase, serum alkaline phosphatase, and serum bilirubin, as well as an increase in protein levels. When compared to the CCl_4-treated group, the thiopentone-induced sleeping period was also reduced in the PNK-treated mice. Because of its antioxidant impact on hepatocytes, it can be assumed that PNK protects hepatocytes from CCl_4-induced liver damage [165].

Rohitakarista is an Ayurvedic polyherbal (Table **2**) hepatoprotective medication [166]. The hepatoprotective activity of Rohitakarista against carbon tetrachloride-induced hepatotoxicity in rats was studied. Rohitakarista treatment reduced CCl_4-induced hepatic architectural changes and preserved liver tissue from necrotic, fatty, and degenerative changes. Rohitakarista's hepatoprotective activity is ascribed to its herbal ingredients, which contain extremely effective antioxidant and hepatoprotective phytoconstituents, and their combined synergistic action helps regulate liver function and cure complex liver illnesses [167].

Anil U. T. studied the hepatoprotective activity of a polyherbal formulation containing spray-dried aqueous extracts of *Andrographis paniculata* Nees. (Acanthaceae), *Phyllanthus niruri* Linn. (Euphorbiaceae), and *Phyllanthus emblica* Linn. (Euphorbiaceae) against paracetamol, carbon tetrachloride (CCl_4), and ethanol-induced hepatic damage in rats. Serum marker enzymes such as SGOT, SGPT, ALP, direct bilirubin (DB), and lactate dehydrogenase were used to assess Polyherbal formulation. The biochemical measurements were also supported by histology examinations. The standard medication was silymarin PHF (100 and 200 mg/kg p.o.) significantly reduced the rise of SGPT, SGOT,

ALP, DB, and LDH caused by paracetamol, CCl_4, and ethanol. In comparison to the toxicant group, a comparative histological analysis of the liver revealed almost normal architecture. The combined action of all plant extracts and their phytoconstituents suggests that PHF's hepatoprotective actions may be effective for liver protection [168].

Arti Gupta *et al.* developed Polyherbal formulations by combining three bioactive fractionated extracts of *Butea monosperma, Bauhinia variegata*, and *Ocimum gratissimum* for the treatment of liver disorders, based on traditional and medical knowledge and tested for hepatoprotective activity using a paracetamol-induced liver damage model in rats. At 100 mg/kg, a biochemical marker revealed enhanced results for polyherbal tablet formulation. Polyherbal tablet formulation has a powerful hepatoprotective substance, which is thought to be a flavone enriched in the polyherbal formulation and could be used in clinical settings to treat paracetamol-induced liver damage [169].

The Livshis polyherbal formulation is used in Ayurvedic medicine (Table **2**) to treat hepatic diseases in the Indian state of West Bengal. Livshis was given orally at doses ranging from 25 to 3200 mg/kg body weight in order to assess its acute toxicity. This study looked at the hepatoprotective effect of the polyherbal formulation Livshis in CCl_4-induced hepatotoxicity in male albino rats, as well as the formulation's toxicity. The active Phyto-ingredients in Livshis aid in stabilising hepatocyte plasma membranes and sustaining their transport function. By shielding serum marker enzyme activity, the formulation also aids in the healing of hepatic tissue. At the oral doses examined, the formulation was well tolerated, with no symptoms of clinical toxicity or evidence of hepatic, reno, or hematotoxicity [170].

In carbon tetrachloride-induced hepatotoxicity, hepatoprotective polyherbal formulation Livergen (Table **2**) is tested for hepatoprotective efficacy. The activities of SGOT, SGPT, ALP, Cholesterol, Bilirubin, and Total protein were estimated to assess liver function. The results of the investigation show that the formulation has a lot of action. The Polyherbal formulation Livergen resulted in a substantial drop in SGOT, SGPT, ALP, Cholesterol, and Bilirubin enzyme levels, as well as a significant increase in Total protein enzyme levels (P 0.01). Its application as a hepatoprotective agent is complicated by its polyherbal composition [171].

Himoliv (HV) (Table **2**) was tested in rats with hepatotoxicity caused by carbon tetrachloride or paracetamol. A single dosage of carbon tetrachloride (CCl_4, 1 ml/kg, 50 percent v/v with olive oil, s.c.) or paracetamol (PC, 1 g/kg, p.o.) was used to induce liver necrosis. The elevated level of Serum glutamate oxaloacetate transaminase (SGOT), serum glutamate pyruvate transaminase (SGPT), serum alkaline phosphatase (ALP), hepatic thiobarbituric acid reacting substances (TBARS), and superoxide dismutase (SOD) all showed signs of liver injury. CCl_4 or PC-induced increases of SGOT, SGPT, ALP, and TBARS were considerably (P 0.001) reduced by HV pre-treatment (0.5 and 1.0 ml/kg, p.o.), whereas the reduced concentration of SOD owing to CCl_4 or PC was reversed. Similar outcomes were shown with silymarin (25 mg/ kg, p.o.), a well-known hepatoprotective medication [172].

Hepax is employed as a hepato-stimulant, hepatoprotective, and hepato-regenerative agent, and it has a wide range of applications in the treatment of liver disease (Table **2**). Hepatoprotective effect of Hepax was investigated in rats exposed to three experimentally produced hepatotoxicity models: carbon tetrachloride (CCl_4), paracetamol, and thioacetamide. Hepatotoxins (CCl_4, paracetamol, and thioacetamide) caused severe morphological, biochemical, and histological changes in experimental animals' livers. Pre-treatment with Hepax provided significant protection against hepatic damage by keeping morphological parameters (liver weight and liver weight to organ weight ratio) within normal ranges and normalizing elevated levels of biochemical parameters (SGPT, SGOT, ALP, and total bilirubin), as evidenced by histopathological findings. Hepax has a highly significant hepatoprotective impact on the liver of all three experimental animal models at 100 and 200 mg/kg, p.o [173].

Muhammad Fiaz *et al.* tested the hepatoprotective effects of a polyherbal formulation in female rabbits. In animals with hepatic damage caused by paracetamol (PCM), the herbal formulation was utilized alone and in conjunction with ascorbic acid (AsAc). The Polyherbal Formulation is made up of parts from four different medicinal plants: *Zingiber officinale* (Ginger), *Peganum harmala* (Wild Rue), and *Cassia angustifolia* (Senna). PHF was an effective hepatoprotective regimen in mice administered with high doses of paracetamol [174].

In human liver HepG2 cells, the hepatoprotective effect of BV-7310 was studied against alcohol-induced damage (Table **2**). In these cells, ethanol treatment (120 mM for 48 hours) resulted in significant toxicity (about 42%), and incubation with BV-7310 reduced ethanol-induced cell death in a dose-dependent manner. When compared to the vehicle-treated group, both oral dosages of BV-7310 (250 and 500 mg/kg body weight) protected against alcohol-induced weight loss and dramatically improved high liver enzyme levels. Thus, BV-7310 protects against alcohol-induced toxicity in both in vitro and in vivo models, suggesting that it could be useful in the treatment of Alcoholic liver disease (ALD) and other disorders that produce liver toxicity [175].

·P. M. Dandagi *et al.* investigated the hepatoprotective effect of extracts from *Ferula asafoetida, Momordica charantia* Linn, and *Nardostachys jatamansi* against experimental hepatotoxicity. Compared to LIV-52, polyherbal suspensions were produced using extracts with considerable activity and assessed for physicochemical and hepatoprotective effects. The hepatoprotective effect of petroleum ether (60-80°), chloroform, benzene, ethanol, and aqueous extracts of *Ferula asafoetida, Momordica charantia* Linn, and *Nardostachys jatamansi* against carbon tetrachloride-induced liver damage in Wistar rats was investigated. Using the trituration method, a suspending agent and various excipients were used to make polyherbal suspensions. By lowering increased blood enzymes levels such as glutamate oxaloacetate transaminase, glutamate pyruvate transaminase, and alkaline phosphatase, the formulation has been demonstrated to have a strong hepatoprotective impact. Histopathological evaluation of liver sections was used to supplement these analytical findings. Treatment with formulation improves recovery from carbon tetrachloride-induced hepatotoxicity, according to research. The formulation (containing chloroform, petroleum ether, and aqueous extracts of *Ferula asafoetida*, petroleum ether and ethanol extracts of *Momordica charantia* Linn., and petroleum ether and ethanol extracts of *Nardostachys jatamansi*) showed significant hepatoprotective activity, which could be due to the combined effect of all these extracts [176].

Shilpa N. Patere *et al.* studied the effects of oral treatment with Normeta® (2 ml and 4 ml/kg) on hepatic damage induced by alcohol (10–30%), thermally oxidized oil (polyunsaturated fatty acids) (15 percent of diet), and carbonyl iron (1.5–2% of diet) in rats for 30 days (Blood alcohol levels were maintained between 150 and 350 mg/dl). Normeta® (Table **2**) has antioxidant and metal chelating activity, according to in vitro experiments with 1, 1-diphenyl-2-picrylhydrazyl (DPPH), nitric oxide, and ferric chloride (Fe^{+3} ions). Alcohol, polyunsaturated fatty acids, and iron supplementation increased serum iron levels and serum glutamate pyruvate transaminase while decreasing serum proteins. It was also linked to increased lipid peroxidation (thiobarbituric acid reactive chemicals) and disruption of the liver's antioxidant defense mechanism, as well as lower body weight and a higher liver-to-body-weight ratio. Oral Normeta® combined with alcohol, polyunsaturated fatty acids, and iron reduced serum iron, serum glutamate pyruvate transaminase and raised serum protein levels. The activities of antioxidant enzymes superoxide dismutase and catalase were raised while the levels of liver thiobarbituric acid reactive compounds were lowered. There was also an improvement in body weight and the liver-to-body weight ratio. Normeta® had impacts on physical-metabolic parameters that were comparable to silymarin. This suggests that Normeta® is effective in reducing the severity of hepatotoxicity [177].

The hepatoprotective efficacy of polyherbal formulations, including hydro alcoholic extract of *Tinospora cordifolia* and ethanol extracts of *Boerhavia diffusa, Phyllanthus amarus, Euphorbia hirta,* and *Wedelia chinesis* was studied by V. Sivakumar *et al.* The hepatoprotective effects of three different herbal formulations from diverse medicinal plant extracts were tested in rats after paracetamol-induced liver injury. To induce hepatotoxicity, a single dosage of paracetamol (3g/kg, p.o) was given. For 8 days, Formulation (200mg/kg, p.o) and silymarin (25mg/kg, p.o) were given once daily. The degree of hepatoprotection was assessed using morphological markers such as color changes and the weight of the liver. Serum glutamate oxaloacetate transaminase (SGOT), serum glutamate pyruvate transaminase (SGPT), serum alkaline phosphatase (SALP), bilirubin, and plasma protein biochemical markers were investigated. The histopathological parameters of histological alterations in the liver architecture, such as hepatic lobule architecture, liver cell swelling, fatty changes, localized necrosis, inflammatory cell infiltration around portal sites, kupffer cell hyperplasia, and so on. As a functional parameter, the functional parameters of pentobarbitone sleeping time were used. In experimental animals, polyherbal formulation had considerable hepatoprotective properties against paracetamol-induced liver injury [178].

CONCLUSION

The liver is an important organ that aids in the metabolism and elimination of xenobiotics from the body. Liver injury or malfunction is a serious public health issue that affects not only doctors and nurses but also the pharmaceutical business and drug regulatory bodies. Various harmful compounds (antibiotics, chemotherapeutic drugs, carbon tetrachloride (CCl_4), thioacetamide (TAA), *etc.*), excessive alcohol consumption, and microbes that cause liver cell damage are well studied. In this scenario, the current synthetic medications to treat liver problems promote more liver damage. As a result, herbal drugs have grown in popularity and are widely used. For a long time, herbal remedies have been utilized to treat liver problems. There are a variety of herbal preparations on the market. Herbal and traditional botanical preparations have been utilized for the treatment of numerous ailments and diseases since ancient times. Several medicinal plants have anticancer, cardiotonic, diuretic, antiarrhythmic, and other therapeutic properties in addition to hepatoprotective properties. The goal of this review is to compile information on promising phytochemicals from medicinal plants that have been investigated in hepatotoxicity models utilizing cutting-edge scientific methods. Herb-based treatments for liver problems have been used in India for a long time and have been popularised by major pharmaceutical companies all over the world. Despite their widespread use, herbal medicines in general, and herbal medications for liver illnesses in particular, are still considered unsuitable therapy options for liver ailments. Natural therapies for liver disease treatment have a long history, dating back to Ayurvedic medicine and extending to Chinese, European, and other traditional medicine systems. Hepatoprotective activity has been claimed for a variety of plants and preparations. New hepatoprotective plants are important for the development of medications that are less expensive, have fewer side effects, are more potent, and enable effective hepatoprotection and immune response treatments to be developed. The goal of this review is to compile data from published studies on promising phytochemicals from medicinal plants that have been examined in hepatotoxicity models. Herbal medicines are becoming increasingly popular around the world, with ethnobotanicals being used by at least a quarter of patients with liver problems. To unravel the mysteries concealed in the plants, more efforts should be put into methodical scientific examination for their safety and efficacy by subjecting them to rigorous preclinical investigations followed by clinical trials. This method will aid in the investigation of the true therapeutic potential of these natural pharmacotherapeutic substances, as well as the standardization of dosing regimens based on evidence-based discoveries, allowing them to become more than a fad. Many herbal formulations are available to help with health, symptom relief, and illness cure. The majority of these products, on the other hand, lack scientific pharmacological confirmation. Several herbs showed hepatoprotective/curative benefits in the laboratory or higher animal hepatotoxicity models, indicating that a clinical study is warranted. Most herbal formulations cannot be advised for the treatment of liver problems due to a lack of scientifically supported pharmacological data. In this review article, we have attempted to gather and consolidate information on a few hepatoprotective natural items that will be valuable to society as it moves into the realm of alternative medicine. In the near future, a more comprehensive assessment of numerous herbal products available as hepato-protectants overseas will be published.

REFERENCES

[1]   Ilyas, U.; Katare, D.P.; Aeri, V.; Naseef, P.P. A review on hepatoprotective and immunomodulatory herbal plants. *Pharmacogn. Rev.,* **2016**, *10*(19), 66-70.
        [http://dx.doi.org/10.4103/0973-7847.176544] [PMID: 27041876]

[2]   Almazroo, O.A.; Miah, M.K.; Venkataramanan, R. Drug metabolism in the liver. *Clin. Liver Dis.,* **2017**, *21*(1), 1-20.
        [http://dx.doi.org/10.1016/j.cld.2016.08.001] [PMID: 27842765]

[3]   Miller, L.L.; Bale, W.F. Synthesis of all plasma protein fractions except gamma globulins by the liver: The use of zone electrophoresis and lysine-epsilon-C14 to define the plasma proteins synthesized by the isolated perfused liver. *J. Exp. Med.,* **1954**, *99*(2), 125-132.
        [http://dx.doi.org/10.1084/jem.99.2.125] [PMID: 13130789]

[4]   Bechmann, L.P.; Hannivoort, R.A.; Gerken, G.; Hotamisligil, G.S.; Trauner, M.; Canbay, A. The interaction of hepatic lipid and glucose metabolism in liver diseases. *J. Hepatol.,* **2012**, *56*(4), 952-964.
        [http://dx.doi.org/10.1016/j.jhep.2011.08.025] [PMID: 22173168]

[5]   Timens, W.; Kamps, W.A.; Rozeboom-Uiterwijk, T.; Poppema, S. Haemopoiesis in human fetal and embryonic liver. Immunohistochemical determination in B5-fixed paraffin-embedded tissues. *Virchows Arch. A Pathol. Anat. Histopathol.,* **1990,** *416*(5), 429-436.
[http://dx.doi.org/10.1007/BF01605149] [PMID: 2107630]

[6]   Nguyen-Lefebvre, A.T.; Horuzsko, A. Kupffer cell metabolism and function. *Journal of Enzymology and Metabolism.,* **2015,** *1*(1), 101.
[PMID: 26937490]

[7]   Memon, N.; Weinberger, B.I.; Hegyi, T.; Aleksunes, L.M. Inherited disorders of bilirubin clearance. *Pediatr. Res.,* **2016,** *79*(3), 378-386.
[http://dx.doi.org/10.1038/pr.2015.247] [PMID: 26595536]

[8]   Functions of liver. https://mysciencesquad.weebly.com/d3-functions-of-the-liver.html

[9]   Shneider, Benjamin; Sherman, L.; Philip, M. Pediatric gastrointestinal disease. *Connecticut,* **2008,** 751.

[10]   Wang, F.S.; Fan, J.G.; Zhang, Z.; Gao, B.; Wang, H.Y. The global burden of liver disease: The major impact of China. *Hepatology,* **2014,** *60*(6), 2099-2108. a
[http://dx.doi.org/10.1002/hep.27406] [PMID: 25164003]

[11]   Fatma, N.; Upadhyay, R.P. Euphorbia nivulia buch. ham.a boon for jaundice (A Case Study). *Annals of Plant Sciences.,* **2015,** *4*(6), 1137-1139.

[12]   Akila, M.; Prasanna, G. Hepatoprotective Effect of *Indigofera Linnael.* on carbon tetrachloride induced wistar albino rats. *I. RES. J. PHARMA.,* **2014,** *5*(5), 392-395.
[http://dx.doi.org/10.7897/2230-8407.050581]

[13]   Pandit, A.; Sachdeva, T.; Bafna, P. Drug-induced hepatotoxicity: A Review. *J. Appl. Pharm. Sci.,* **2012,** (5), 233-243.

[14]   Ostapowicz, G.; Fontana, R.J.; Schiødt, F.V.; Larson, A.; Davern, T.J.; Han, S.H.; McCashland, T.M.; Shakil, A.O.; Hay, J.E.; Hynan, L.; Crippin, J.S.; Blei, A.T.; Samuel, G.; Reisch, J.; Lee, W.M. Results of a prospective study of acute liver failure at 17 tertiary care centers in the United States. *Ann. Intern. Med.,* **2002,** *137*(12), 947-954.
[http://dx.doi.org/10.7326/0003-4819-137-12-200212170-00007] [PMID: 12484709]

[15]   Bedi, O.; Bijjem, K.R.V.; Kumar, P.; Gauttam, V. Herbal induced hepatoprotection and hepatotoxicity: A critical review. *Indian J. Physiol. Pharmacol.,* **2016,** *60*(1), 6-21.
[PMID: 29953177]

[16]   McMahon, BJ. Epidemiology and natural history of hepatitis B. *Semin Liver Dis.,* **2005,** *25* 1, 3-8.

[17]   Ekaidem, I S; Akpan, H D; Usoh, I F; Etim, OE; Ebong, PE . Effect of ethanolic extract of azadirachta indica leaves on lipid peroxidation and serum lipids of diabetic wistar rats. *Acta Biological Szegedensis.,* **2007,** *51*(1), 17-20.

[18]   Anand, K.; Lal, U.R. Hepatitis and medicinal plants. *RE:view,* **2016,** *5*(6), 408-415.

[19]   Jannu, V.; Baddam, P.G.; Boorgula, A.K.; Jambula, S.R. A review on hepatoprotective plant plants. *Inter J Drug Development Res.,* **2012,** *4*(3), 1-8.

[20]   Sivakrishnan, S. Liver diseases :An overview. *World J. Pharm. Pharm. Sci.,* **2019,** *8*(1), 1385.

[21]   Chattopadhyay, R.R. Possible mechanism of hepatoprotective activity of *Azadirachta indica* leaf extract: part II. *J. Ethnopharmacol.,* **2003,** *89*(2-3), 217-219.
[http://dx.doi.org/10.1016/j.jep.2003.08.006] [PMID: 14611885]

[22]   Adewusi, E.A.; Afolayan, A.J. A review of natural products with hepatoprotective activity. *J. Med. Plants Res.,* **2010,** *4*(13), 1318-1334.

[23]   Deshwal, N.; Sharma, A.K.; Sharma, P. Review on hepatoprotective plants. *Int. J. Pharm. Sci. Rev. Res.,* **2011,** *7*, 15-26.

[24]　Jannu, V.; Baddam, P.G.; Boorgula, A.K.; Jambula, S.R. A review on hepatoprotective plants. *Inter J Drug Development Res.,* **2012**, *4*(3), 1-8.

[25]　Handa, S.S.; Sharma, A.; Chakarborty, K.K. Natural Products and plants as liver protecting drugs. *Fitoterapia,* **1986**, *57*(5), 307-351.

[26]　Panda, S.; Kar, A. Periplogenin-3-O- -D-glucopyranosyl -(1-->6)- -D-glucopyaranosyl- -(1-->4) -- -cymaropyranoside, isolated from Aegle marmelos protects doxorubicin induced cardiovascular problems and hepatotoxicity in rats. *Cardiovasc. Ther.,* **2009**, *27*(2), 108-116.
[http://dx.doi.org/10.1111/j.1755-5922.2009.00078.x] [PMID: 19426248]

[27]　Seema, P.V.; Sudha, B.; Padayatti, P.S.; Abraham, A.; Raghu, K.G.; Paulose, C.S. Kinetic studies of purified malate dehydrogenase in liver of streptozotocin-diabetic rats and the effect of leaf extract of *Aegle marmelose* (L.) Correa ex Roxb. *Indian J. Exp. Biol.,* **1996**, *34*(6), 600-602.
[PMID: 8792652]

[28]　Singh, R.; Rao, H. Hepatoprotective effect of the pulp/seed of Aegle marmelos correa ex Roxb against carbon tetrachloride induced liver damage in rats. *I. J. Green Pharmacy,* **2008**, *2*(4), 232.
[http://dx.doi.org/10.4103/0973-8258.44740]

[29]　Baliga, M.S.; Thilakchand, K.R.; Rai, M.P.; Rao, S.; Venkatesh, P. *Aegle marmelos* (L.) Correa (Bael) and its phytochemicals in the treatment and prevention of cancer. *Integr. Cancer Ther.,* **2013**, *12*(3), 187-196.
[http://dx.doi.org/10.1177/1534735412451320] [PMID: 23089553]

[30]　Sherwood, E.R.; Toliver-Kinsky, T. Mechanisms of the inflammatory response. *Baillieres. Best Pract. Res. Clin. Anaesthesiol.,* **2004**, *18*(3), 385-405.
[http://dx.doi.org/10.1016/j.bpa.2003.12.002] [PMID: 15212335]

[31]　Rathee, D.; Kamboj, A.; Sidhu, S. Augmentation of hepatoprotective potential of aegle marmelos in combination with piperine in carbon tetrachloride model in wistar rats. *Chem. Cent. J.,* **2018**, *12*(1), 94.
[http://dx.doi.org/10.1186/s13065-018-0463-9] [PMID: 30123925]

[32]　Choudhury, B.R.; Poddar, M.K. Andrographolide and kalmegh (*Andrographis paniculata*) extract: *In vivo* and *in vitro* effect on hepatic lipid peroxidation. *Methods Find. Exp. Clin. Pharmacol.,* **1984**, *6*(9), 481-485.
[PMID: 6513681]

[33]　Rana, A.C.; Avadhoot, Y. Hepatoprotective effects of *Andrographis paniculata* against carbon tetrachloride-induced liver damage. *Arch. Pharm. Res.,* **1991**, *14*(1), 93-95.
[http://dx.doi.org/10.1007/BF02857822] [PMID: 10319129]

[34]　Handa, S.S.; Sharma, A. Hepatoprotective activity of andrographolide from *Andrographis paniculata* against carbontetrachloride. *Indian J. Med. Res.,* **1990**, *92*, 276-283.
[PMID: 2228074]

[35]　Verma, V.K.; Sarwa, K.K.; Kumar, A.; Zaman, M.K. Comparison of hepatoprotective activity of *Swertia chirayita* and *Andrographis paniculata* plant of North–East India against CCl$_4$ induced hepatotoxic rats. *J. Pharm. Res.,* **2013**, *7*(7), 647-653.
[http://dx.doi.org/10.1016/j.jopr.2013.07.008]

[36]　Handa, S.S.; Sharma, A. Hepatoprotective activity of andrographolide against galactosamine & paracetamol intoxication in rats. *Indian J. Med. Res.,* **1990**, *92*, 284-292.
[PMID: 2228075]

[37]　Kapil, A.; Koul, I.B.; Banerjee, S.K.; Gupta, B.D. Antihepatotoxic effects of major diterpenoid constituents of andrographis paniculata. *Biochem. Pharmacol.,* **1993**, *46*(1), 182-185.
[http://dx.doi.org/10.1016/0006-2952(93)90364-3] [PMID: 8347130]

[38]　Ilyasnasim, S.M.; Adnan, J. hepatoprotective effect of garlic and milk thistle (silymarin) in isoniazid induces hepatotoxicity in rats. *Biomedica,* **2011**, *27*(2), 166-170.

[39]   Obioha, U.E.; Suru, S.M.; Ola-Mudathir, K.F.; Faremi, T.Y. Hepatoprotective potentials of onion and garlic extracts on cadmium-induced oxidative damage in rats. *Biol. Trace Elem. Res.,* **2009**, *129*(1-3), 143-156.
[http://dx.doi.org/10.1007/s12011-008-8276-7] [PMID: 19082532]

[40]   Ghorbel, H.; Feki, I.; Friha, I.; Khabir, A.M.; Boudawara, T.; Boudawara, M.; Sayadi, S. Biochemical and histological liver changes occurred after iron supplementation and possible remediation by garlic consumption. *Endocrine,* **2011**, *40*(3), 462-471.
[http://dx.doi.org/10.1007/s12020-011-9483-0] [PMID: 21553301]

[41]   Patrick-Iwuanyanwu, K.C.; Wegwu, M.O.; Ayalogu, E.O. Prevention of CCl4-induced liver damage by ginger, garlic and vitamin E. *Pak. J. Biol. Sci.,* **2007**, *10*(4), 617-621.
[http://dx.doi.org/10.3923/pjbs.2007.617.621] [PMID: 19069545]

[42]   El-Beshbishy, H.A. Aqueous garlic extract attenuates hepatitis and oxidative stress induced by galactosamine/lipoploysaccharide in rats. *Phytother. Res.,* **2008**, *22*(10), 1372-1379.
[http://dx.doi.org/10.1002/ptr.2505] [PMID: 18570225]

[43]   Park, E.Y.; Ki, S.H.; Ko, M.S.; Kim, C.W.; Lee, M.H.; Lee, Y.S.; Kim, S.G. Garlic oil and DDB, comprised in a pharmaceutical composition for the treatment of patients with viral hepatitis, prevents acute liver injuries potentiated by glutathione deficiency in rats. *Chem. Biol. Interact.,* **2005**, *155*(1-2), 82-96.
[http://dx.doi.org/10.1016/j.cbi.2005.04.006] [PMID: 15950962]

[44]   Price, K.R.; Rhodes, M.J.C. Analysis of the major flavonol glycosides present in four varieties of onion (*Allium cepa*) and changes in composition resulting from autolysis. *J. Sci. Food Agric.,* **1997**, *74*(3), 331-339.
[http://dx.doi.org/10.1002/(SICI)1097-0010(199707)74:3<331::AID-JSFA806>3.0.CO;2-C]

[45]   Ozougwu, J.C.; Nwachi, U.E.; Eyo, J.E. Comparative hypolipidaemic effects of *Allium cepa, Allium sativum* and *Zingiber officinale* aqueous extracts on alloxan-induced diabetic Rattus novergicus. *Biol. Res.,* **2008**, *6*(2), 384-391.

[46]   Eyo, J.E.; Ozougwu, J.C.; Echi, P.C. Hypoglycaemic effects of *Allium cepa, Allium sativum* and *Zingiber officinale* aqueous extracts on alloxan-induced diabetic *Rattus novergicus. Med J Islam World Acad of Sci.,* **2011**, *19*, 121-126.

[47]   Ozougwu, J.C. Anti-diabetic effects of *Allium cepa* (Onions) aqueous extracts on alloxan-induced diabetic Rattus novergicus. *J. Med. Plants Res.,* **2011**, *5*(7), 1134-1139.

[48]   Ozougwu, J C; Eyo, J E Hepatoprotective effects of *Allium cepa (onoin)* extracts against paracetamol induced liver damage in rats. *African J Biotech.,* **2014**, *13*(26), 2679-2688.

[49]   Eswar Kumar, K.; Harsha, K.N.; Sudheer, V.; Giri babu, N. *in vitro* antioxidant activity and *in vivo* hepatoprotective activity of aqueous extract of *Allium cepa* bulb in ethanol induced liver damage in Wistar rats. *Food Sci. Hum. Wellness,* **2013**, *2*(3-4), 132-138.
[http://dx.doi.org/10.1016/j.fshw.2013.10.001]

[50]   Ige, S F; Akhigbe, R E; Adewale, A A P Effect of *Allium cepa (onion)* extract on cadmium Induced nephrotoxicity in rats. *Kidney Res J.,* **2011**, *1*(1), 41-47.

[51]   Lee, K.J.; Kim, D.S.; Seo, E.S. Hepatoprotective effects of *Allium cepa* L. extract on acetaminophen induced liver damage in mice. *Food Sci. Biotechnol.,* **2003**, *12*(6), 612-616.

[52]   Kirtikar, K R; Basu, B D Indian medicinal plants. Periodic expert book agency: new delhi, **1991**; pp. 478-482.

[53]   Sen, P.; Mediratta, P.K.; Ray, A. Effects of azadirachta indica a juss on some biochemical, immunological and visceral parameters in normal and stressed rats. *Indian J. Exp. Biol.,* **1992**, *30*(12), 1170-1175.
[PMID: 1294481]

[54]   Patel, P.M.; Gohil, T.A.; Malavia, S.V.; Bhalodia, Y.S.; Shah, G.B. Comparative *in vitro* hepatoprotective activity of different extracts of *Azadiracta indica* leaves. *J. Pharm. Res.,* **2012**, *5*, 2122-2125.

[55]   Gomase, P.V.; Rangari, V.D.; Verma, P.R. Phytochemical evaluation and hepatoprotective activity of fresh juice of young stem (tender) bark of *Azadiracta indica.* A. juss. *Int. J. Pharma Sci.,* **2011**, *3*(2), 55-59.

[56]   Chattopadhyay, R.R.; Sarkar, S.K.; Ganguly, S.; Banerjee, R.N.; Basu, T.K.; Mukherjee, A. hepatoprotective activity of azadirachta indica leaves on paracetamol induced hepatic damage in rats. *Indian J. Exp. Biol.,* **1992**, *30*(8), 738-740.
[PMID: 1459654]

[57]   Tahmasebi, M.; Sadeghi, H.; Nazem, H.; Kokhdan, E.P.; Omidifar, N. Hepatoprotective effects of *Berberis vulgaris* leaf extract on carbon tetrachloride-induced hepatotoxicity in rats. *J. Educ. Health Promot.,* **2018**, *7*, 147.
[PMID: 30596119]

[58]   Anca, H; Cristina, P; Aurel, A; Miruna, S Hepatoprotective effects of *Berberis vulgaris L.* extract/β cyclodextrin on carbon tetrachloride–induced acute toxicity in miceInt. *J Mol Sci.,* **2012**, *13*(7), 9014-9034.

[59]   Hwang, J.M.; Wang, C.J.; Chou, F.P.; Tseng, T-H.; Hsieh, Y-S.; Lin, W-L.; Chu, C-Y. Inhibitory effect of berberine on tert-butyl hydroperoxide-induced oxidative damage in rat liver. *Arch. Toxicol.,* **2002**, *76*(11), 664-670.
[http://dx.doi.org/10.1007/s00204-002-0351-9] [PMID: 12415430]

[60]   Fallah, H.; Zarrei, M.; Ziai, M. The effects of *Taraxacum officinale* L. and *Berberis vulgaris* L. root extracts on carbon tetrachloride induced liver toxicity in rats. *Faslnamah-i Giyahan-i Daruyi,* **2010**, *9*(33), 45-52.

[61]   Mishra, S.; Aeri, V.; Gaur, P.K.; Jachak, S.M. Phytochemical, therapeutic, and ethnopharmacological overview for a traditionally important herb: Boerhavia diffusa Linn. *BioMed Res. Int.,* **2014**, *2014*, 808302.
[PMID: 24949473]

[62]   Venkatalakshmi, P.; Eazhisai, V.D.; Netaji, S. Hepatoprotective activity of *Boerhavia diffusa* against paracetamol induced toxicity in rats. *J. Chem. Pharm. Res.,* **2011**, *3*, 229-232.

[63]   Olaleye, M.T.; Akinmoladun, A.C.; Ogunboye, A.A.; Akindahunsi, A.A. Antioxidant activity and hepatoprotective property of leaf extracts of Boerhaavia diffusa Linn against acetaminophen-induced liver damage in rats. *Food Chem. Toxicol.,* **2010**, *48*(8-9), 2200-2205.
[http://dx.doi.org/10.1016/j.fct.2010.05.047] [PMID: 20553784]

[64]   Rawat, A.K.S.; Mehrotra, S.; Tripathi, S.C.; Shome, U. Hepatoprotective activity of *Boerhaavia diffusa* L. roots--a popular Indian ethnomedicine. *J. Ethnopharmacol.,* **1997**, *56*(1), 61-66.
[http://dx.doi.org/10.1016/S0378-8741(96)01507-3] [PMID: 9147255]

[65]   Chakraborti, K.K.; Handa, S.S. Antihepatotoxic investigations of *Boerhaavia diffusa* L. *Indian Drugs.,* **1989**, *27*, 161-166.

[66]   Singh, V.; Pandey, R.P. Medicinal plant lore of the tribals of eastern Rajasthan. *J. Econ. Taxon. Bot.,* **1980**, *1*, 137-147.

[67]   Gopal, G.V.; Shah, G.L. Some folk medicinal plants used for jaundice in Gujarat, India. *J. Res. Educ. Indian Med.,* **1985**, *4*, 44-49.

[68]   Shameela, S.; Shamshad, S.; Indira, P.A.; John, P.M.; Lakshmi, D.K. Hypolipidemic and anti inflammatory activity of *Boerhaavia diffusa* in isoproterenol-induced myocardial infarcted rats. *Int J Pharm Bio Sci.,* **2015**, *6*, 1-10.

[69]   Bhakta, T.; Banerjee, S.; Mandal, S.C.; Maity, T.K.; Saha, B.P.; Pal, M. Hepatoprotective activity of

cassia fistula leaf extract. *Phytomedicine,* **2001**, *8*(3), 220-224.
[http://dx.doi.org/10.1078/0944-7113-00029] [PMID: 11417916]

[70]   Xie, Q.; Guo, F.F.; Zhou, W. Protective effects of cassia seed ethanol extract against carbon tetrachloride-induced liver injury in mice. *Acta Biochim. Pol.,* **2012**, *59*(2), 265-270.
[http://dx.doi.org/10.18388/abp.2012_2149] [PMID: 22693685]

[71]   Pradeep, K.; Raj Mohan, C.V.; Gobianand, K.; Karthikeyan, S. Protective effect of *Cassia fistula* Linn. on diethylnitrosamine induced hepatocellular damage and oxidative stress in ethanol pretreated rats. *Biol. Res.,* **2010**, *43*(1), 113-125.
[http://dx.doi.org/10.4067/S0716-97602010000100013] [PMID: 21157638]

[72]   Kalantari, H.; Jalali, M.; Jalali, A.; Mahdavinia, M.; Salimi, A.; Juhasz, B.; Tosaki, A.; Gesztelyi, R. Protective effect of *Cassia fistula* fruit extract against bromobenzene-induced liver injury in mice. *Hum. Exp. Toxicol.,* **2011**, *30*(8), 1039-1044.
[http://dx.doi.org/10.1177/0960327110386256] [PMID: 20930029]

[73]   Viswanatha Swamy, A.H.; Kulkarni, R.V.; Thippeswamy, A.H.M.; Koti, B.C.; Gore, A. Evaluation of hepatoprotective activity of *Cissus quadrangularis* stem extract against isoniazid-induced liver damage in rats. *Indian J. Pharmacol.,* **2010**, *42*(6), 397-400.
[http://dx.doi.org/10.4103/0253-7613.71920] [PMID: 21189914]

[74]   Swamy, A.H.; Kulkarni, R.V.; Koti, B.C.; Gadad, P.C.; Thippeswamy, A.H.M.; Gore, A. Hepatoprotective effect of *Cissus quadrangularis* stem extract against rifampicin-induced hepatotoxicity in rats. *Indian J. Pharm. Sci.,* **2012**, *74*(2), 183-187.
[http://dx.doi.org/10.4103/0250-474X.103859] [PMID: 23326004]

[75]   Chidambaram J, Venkatraman CA. Cissus quadrangularis stem alleviates insulin resistance, oxidative injury and fatty liver disease in rats fed high fat plus fructose diet. *Food and chemical toxicology: an international journal published for the British Industrial Biological Research Association.* **2010**; 48(8-9): 2021–2029.

[76]   Jainu, M.; Shyamala Devi, C.S. Attenuation of neutrophil infiltration and proinflammatory cytokines by *Cissus quadrangularis*: a possible prevention against gastric ulcerogenesis. *J. Herb. Pharmacother.,* **2005**, *5*(3), 33-42.
[http://dx.doi.org/10.1080/J157v05n03_04] [PMID: 16520296]

[77]   Pandey, G.S. Dravyaguna vijnana. Krishnadas Academy: Varanasi, India, **2002**; 1, pp. 737-746.

[78]   Mu-En, W; Yi-C, C Curcumin protects against thioacetamide-induced hepatic fibrosis by attenuating the inflammatory response and inducing apoptosis of damaged hepatocytes. *Nutr Biochem,* **2012**, *23*(10), 1352-1366.

[79]   Salama, S.M.; Abdulla, M.A.; AlRashdi, A.S.; Ismail, S.; Alkiyumi, S.S.; Golbabapour, S. Hepatoprotective effect of ethanolic extract of *Curcuma longa* on thioacetamide induced liver cirrhosis in rats. *BMC Complement. Altern. Med.,* **2013**, *13*(1), 56.
[http://dx.doi.org/10.1186/1472-6882-13-56] [PMID: 23496995]

[80]   Tabassum, N; Agarwal, S S Hepatoprotective activity of *Eclipta alba* hassk. against paracetamol-induced hepatocellular damage in mice. *Experimental medicine.,* **2004**, *11*(4), 278-280.

[81]   Saxena, A.K.; Singh, B.; Anand, K.K. Hepatoprotective effects of *Eclipta alba* on subcellular levels in rats. *J. Ethnopharmacol.,* **1993**, *40*(3), 155-161.
[http://dx.doi.org/10.1016/0378-8741(93)90063-B] [PMID: 8145570]

[82]   Lal, V.K.; Kumar, A.; Kumar, P.; Yadav, K.S. Screening of leaves and roots of *Eclipta alba* for hepatoprotective activity. *Arch. Appl. Sci. Res.,* **2010**, *2*(1), 86-94.

[83]   Li, C.P.; Li, R.C. An introductory note to ginseng. *Am. J. Chin. Med.,* **1973**, *1*(2), 249-261.
[http://dx.doi.org/10.1142/S0192415X73000279] [PMID: 4359507]

[84]   Attele, A.S.; Wu, J.A.; Yuan, C.S. Ginseng pharmacology: Multiple constituents and multiple actions. *Biochem. Pharmacol.,* **1999**, *58*(11), 1685-1693.

[http://dx.doi.org/10.1016/S0006-2952(99)00212-9] [PMID: 10571242]

[85]   Han, J.Y.; Lee, S.; Yang, J.H.; Kim, S.; Sim, J.; Kim, M.G.; Jeong, T.C.; Ku, S.K.; Cho, I.J.; Ki, S.H. Korean Red Ginseng attenuates ethanol-induced steatosis and oxidative stress via AMPK/Sirt1 activation. *J. Ginseng Res.,* **2015**, *39*(2), 105-115.
[http://dx.doi.org/10.1016/j.jgr.2014.09.001] [PMID: 26045683]

[86]   Park, H.M.; Kim, S.J.; Mun, A.R.; Go, H-K.; Kim, G-B.; Kim, S-Z.; Jang, S-I.; Lee, S-J.; Kim, J-S.; Kang, H-S. Korean red ginseng and its primary ginsenosides inhibit ethanol-induced oxidative injury by suppression of the MAPK pathway in TIB-73 cells. *J. Ethnopharmacol.,* **2012**, *141*(3), 1071-1076.
[http://dx.doi.org/10.1016/j.jep.2012.03.038] [PMID: 22472111]

[87]   Lin, C.F.; Wong, K.L.; Wu, R.S.C.; Huang, T.C.; Liu, C.F. Protection by hot water extract of *Panax notoginseng* on chronic ethanol-induced hepatotoxicity. *Phytother. Res.,* **2003**, *17*(9), 1119-1122.
[http://dx.doi.org/10.1002/ptr.1329] [PMID: 14595601]

[88]   Zhang, Z.L.; Li, Z.J.; Liu, S.K.; Zhou, Y.L. Effect of notoginseng radix on expression quantity of TGF-beta1/ Smads and CTGF mRNA in rats with alcoholic liver disease. *Zhongguo Zhongyao Zazhi,* **2013**, *38*(17), 2859-2862.
[PMID: 24380311]

[89]   Lee, M.H.; Lee, B.H.; Lee, S.; Choi, C. Reduction of hepatitis A virus on FRhK-4 cells treated with Korean red ginseng extract and ginsenosides. *J. Food Sci.,* **2013**, *78*(9), M1412-M1415.
[http://dx.doi.org/10.1111/1750-3841.12205] [PMID: 23931146]

[90]   Ashaa, S.; Tajub, G.; Jayanthic, M. Study of hepatoprotective effect of *Hemidesmus indicus* on paracetamol induced liver damage in rats. *J. Pharm. Res.,* **2011**, *4*(3), 624-626.

[91]   Lakshmi, T.; Rajendran, R. hemidesmus indicus commonly known as indian sarasaparilla-an update. *Int J Pharm Bio Sci.,* **2013**, *4*(4), 397-404.

[92]   Prabakan, M.; Anandan, R.; Devaki, T. Protective effect of *Hemidesmus indicus* against rifampicin and isoniazid-induced hepatotoxicity in rats. *Fitoterapia,* **2000**, *71*(1), 55-59.
[http://dx.doi.org/10.1016/S0367-326X(99)00120-3] [PMID: 11449471]

[93]   Mohana Rao, G.M.; Venkateswararao, C.H.; Rawat, A.K.S.; Pushpangadan, P.; Shirwaikar, A. Antioxidant and antihepatotoxic activities of *Hemidesmus indicus* R. Br. *Acta Pharmaceutica Turcica.,* **2005**, *47*(2), 107-113. b

[94]   Baheti, J.R.; Goyal, R.K.; Shah, G.B. Hepatoprotective activity of *Hemidesmus indicus* R. br. in rats. *Indian J. Exp. Biol.,* **2006**, *44*(5), 399-402.
[PMID: 16708894]

[95]   Saravanan, N.; Nalini, N. Inhibitory effect of *Hemidesmus indicus* and its active principle 2-hydroxy 4-methoxy benzoic acid on ethanol-induced liver injury. *Fundam. Clin. Pharmacol.,* **2007**, *21*(5), 507-514.
[http://dx.doi.org/10.1111/j.1472-8206.2007.00500.x] [PMID: 17868203]

[96]   Lahon, K.; Das, S. Hepatoprotective activity of *Ocimum sanctum* alcoholic leaf extract against paracetamol-induced liver damage in Albino rats. *Pharmacognosy Res.,* **2011**, *3*(1), 13-18.
[http://dx.doi.org/10.4103/0974-8490.79110] [PMID: 21731390]

[97]   Choudhary, P.; Ahmed, S.; Khan, N.A. Herbal plants : A boon for hepatotoxicity. *Asian J. Pharm. Clin. Res.,* **2016**, *9*, 37-40.

[98]   Bhargava, K.P.; Singh, N. Anti-stress activity of *Ocimum sanctum* Linn. *Indian J. Med. Res.,* **1981**, *73*, 443-451.
[PMID: 7275241]

[99]   Akilavalli, N; Radhika, J; Brindha, P . Hepatoprotective activity of *Ocimum sanctum Linn* against lead induced toxicity in albino rats. *Asi j. phar. cli.res.,* **2011**, *4*(2), 54-87.

[100] Chattopadhyay, R.R.; Sarkar, S.K.; Ganguly, S.; Medda, C.; Basu, T.K. Hepatoprotective activity of

ocimum sanctum leaf extract against paracetamol induced hepatic damage in rats. *Indian J. Pharmacol.,* **1992**, *24*, 163-165.

[101] Vidhya Malar, H.L.; Mary Mettilda Bai, S. Hepato-Protective Activity of *Phyllanthus emblica* against paracetamol induced hepatic damage in wister albino rats. *African Journal of Basic & Applied Sciences,* **2009**, *1*(1-2), 21-25.

[102] Tasduq, S.A.; Kaisar, P.; Gupta, D.K.; Kapahi, B.K.; Maheshwari, H.S.; Jyotsna, S.; Johri, R.K.; Maheshwari, H. S. Protective effect of a 50% hydroalcoholic fruit extract *of Emblica officinalis* against anti-tuberculosis drugs induced liver toxicity. *Phytother. Res.,* **2005**, *19*(3), 193-197. [http://dx.doi.org/10.1002/ptr.1631] [PMID: 15934014]

[103] Tasduq, S.A.; Mondhe, D.M.; Gupta, D.K.; Baleshwar, M.; Johri, R.K. Reversal of fibrogenic events in liver by *Emblica officinalis* (fruit), an Indian natural drug. *Biol. Pharm. Bull.,* **2005**, *28*(7), 1304-1306. [http://dx.doi.org/10.1248/bpb.28.1304] [PMID: 15997120]

[104] Haque, R.; Bin-Hafeez, B.; Ahmad, I.; Parvez, S.; Pandey, S.; Raisuddin, S. Protective effects of *Emblica officinalis* Gaertn. in cyclophosphamide-treated mice. *Hum. Exp. Toxicol.,* **2001**, *20*(12), 643-650. [http://dx.doi.org/10.1191/096032701718890568] [PMID: 11936579]

[105] Jose, J.K.; Kuttan, R. Hepatoprotective activity of *Emblica officinalis* and Chyavanaprash. *J. Ethnopharmacol.,* **2000**, *72*(1-2), 135-140. [http://dx.doi.org/10.1016/S0378-8741(00)00219-1] [PMID: 10967464]

[106] Sultana, S.; Ahmed, S.; Sharma, S.; Jahangir, T. *Emblica officinalis* reverses thioacetamide-induced oxidative stress and early promotional events of primary hepatocarcinogenesis. *J. Pharm. Pharmacol.,* **2004**, *56*(12), 1573-1579. [http://dx.doi.org/10.1211/0022357044931] [PMID: 15586980]

[107] Pramyothin, P.; Samosorn, P.; Poungshompoo, S.; Chaichantipyuth, C. The protective effects of *Phyllanthus emblica* Linn. extract on ethanol induced rat hepatic injury. *J. Ethnopharmacol.,* **2006**, *107*(3), 361-364. [http://dx.doi.org/10.1016/j.jep.2006.03.035] [PMID: 16750340]

[108] Verma, R.; Chakraborty, D. Alterations in DNA, RNA and protein contents in liver and kidney of mice treated with ochratoxin and their amelioration by *Emblica officinalis* aqueous extract. *Acta Pol. Pharm.,* **2008**, *65*(1), 3-9. [PMID: 18536167]

[109] Chakraborty, D.; Verma, R. Ameliorative effect of *Emblica officinalis* aqueous extract on ochratoxin-induced lipid peroxidation in the kidney and liver of mice. *Int. J. Occup. Med. Environ. Health,* **2010**, *23*(1), 63-73. [http://dx.doi.org/10.2478/v10001-010-0009-4] [PMID: 20442064]

[110] Sharma, A.; Sharma, M.K.; Kumar, M. Modulatory role of *Emblica officinalis* fruit extract against arsenic induced oxidative stress in Swiss albino mice. *Chem. Biol. Interact.,* **2009**, *180*(1), 20-30. [http://dx.doi.org/10.1016/j.cbi.2009.01.012] [PMID: 19428342]

[111] Reddy, V.D.; Padmavathi, P.; Varadacharyulu, N.Ch. *Emblica officinalis* protects against alcohol-induced liver mitochondrial dysfunction in rats. *J. Med. Food,* **2009**, *12*(2), 327-333. [http://dx.doi.org/10.1089/jmf.2007.0694] [PMID: 19459733]

[112] Sidhu, S.; Pandhi, P.; Malhotra, S.; Vaiphei, K.; Khanduja, K.L. Beneficial effects of *Emblica officinalis* in L-arginine-induced acute pancreatitis in rats. *J. Med. Food,* **2011**, *14*(1-2), 147-155. [http://dx.doi.org/10.1089/jmf.2010.1108] [PMID: 21138365]

[113] Shetty, S.N.; Mengi, S.; Vaidya, R.; Vaidya, A.D. A study of standardized extracts of *Picrorhiza kurroa* Royle ex Benth in experimental nonalcoholic fatty liver disease. *J. Ayurveda Integr. Med.,* **2010**, *1*(3), 203-210. [http://dx.doi.org/10.4103/0975-9476.72622] [PMID: 21547049]

[114] Visen, P.K.; Saraswat, B.; Dhawan, B.N. Curative effect of picroliv on primary cultured rat hepatocytes against different hepatotoxins: An *in vitro* study. Division of Pharmacology, Central Drug Research Institute, Lucknow, UP, India. *J. Pharmacol. Toxicol. Methods,* **1998**, *40*(3), 173-179. [http://dx.doi.org/10.1016/S1056-8719(98)00052-5] [PMID: 10334634]

[115] Santra, A.; Das, S.; Maity, A.; Rao, S.B.; Mazumder, D.N. Prevention of carbon tetrachloride-induced hepatic injury in mice *by Picrorhiza kurrooa*. Department of Gastroenterology, Institute of Post Graduate Medical Education and Research, Calcutta. *Indian J. Gastroenterol.,* **1998**, *17*(1), 6-9. [PMID: 9465504]

[116] Saraswat, B.; Visen, P.K.; Patnaik, G.K.; Dhawan, B.N. Protective effect of picroliv, active constituent of *Picrorhiza kurrooa*, against oxytetracycline induced hepatic damage. ICMR Centre for Advanced Pharmacological Research on Traditional Remedies, Central Drug Research Institute, Lucknow, India. *Indian J. Exp. Biol.,* **1997**, *35*(12), 1302-1305. [PMID: 9567764]

[117] Saller, R.; Meier, R.; Brignoli, R. The use of silymarin in the treatment of liver diseases. *Drugs,* **2001**, *61*(14), 2035-2063. [PMID: 11735632]

[118] Flora, K.; Hahn, M.; Rosen, H.; Benner, K. Milk thistle (*Silybum marianum*) for the therapy of liver disease. *Am. J. Gastroenterol.,* **1998**, *93*(2), 139-143. [http://dx.doi.org/10.1111/j.1572-0241.1998.00139.x] [PMID: 9468229]

[119] Pascual, C.; Gonz, R.; Armesto, J.; Muriel, P. Effect of silymarin and silybinin on oxygen radicals. *Drug Dev. Res.,* **1993**, *29*(1), 73-77. [http://dx.doi.org/10.1002/ddr.430290109]

[120] Pradhan, S.C.; Girish, C. Hepatoprotective herbal drug, silymarin from experimental pharmacology to clinical medicine. *Indian J. Med. Res.,* **2006**, *124*(5), 491-504. [PMID: 17213517]

[121] Jia, J.D.; Bauer, M.; Cho, J.J.; Ruehl, M.; Milani, S.; Boigk, G.; Riecken, E.O.; Schuppan, D. Antifibrotic effect of silymarin in rat secondary biliary fibrosis is mediated by downregulation of procollagen α1(I) and TIMP-1. *J. Hepatol.,* **2001**, *35*(3), 392-398. [http://dx.doi.org/10.1016/S0168-8278(01)00148-9] [PMID: 11592601]

[122] Vargas-Mendoza, N.; Madrigal-Santillán, E.; Morales-González, A.; Esquivel-Soto, J.; Esquivel-Chirino, C.; García-Luna Y González-Rubio, M.; Gayosso-de-Lucio, J.A.; Morales-González, J.A. Hepatoprotective effect of silymarin. *World J. Hepatol.,* **2014**, *6*(3), 144-149. [http://dx.doi.org/10.4254/wjh.v6.i3.144] [PMID: 24672644]

[123] Lin, H.M.; Tseng, H.C.; Wang, C.J.; Lin, J.J.; Lo, C.W.; Chou, F.P. Hepatoprotective effects of Solanum nigrum Linn extract against CCl(4)-induced oxidative damage in rats. *Chem. Biol. Interact.,* **2008**, *171*(3), 283-293. [http://dx.doi.org/10.1016/j.cbi.2007.08.008] [PMID: 18045581]

[124] Hsieh, C.C.; Fang, H.L.; Lina, W.C. Inhibitory effect of *Solanum nigrum* on thioacetamide-induced liver fibrosis in mice. *J. Ethnopharmacol.,* **2008**, *119*(1), 117-121. [http://dx.doi.org/10.1016/j.jep.2008.06.002] [PMID: 18606216]

[125] Doorika, P.; Ananthi, T. Antioxidant and Hepatoprotective properties of *Terminalia arjuna* Bark on Isoniazid Induced Toxicity in Albino rats. *Asian J. Pharm. Tech.,* **2012**, *2*(1), 15-18.

[126] Manna, P.; Sinha, M.; Sil, P.C. Aqueous extract of *Terminalia arjuna* prevents carbon tetrachloride induced hepatic and renal disorders. *BMC Complement. Altern. Med.,* **2006**, *6*(1), 33. [http://dx.doi.org/10.1186/1472-6882-6-33] [PMID: 17010209]

[127] Kavitha, B.T.; Shruthi, S.D.; Rai, S.P.; Ramachandra, Y.L. Phytochemical analysis and hepatoprotective properties of *Tinospora cordifolia* against carbon tetrachloride-induced hepatic damage in rats. *J. Basic Clin. Pharm.,* **2011**, *2*(3), 139-142.

[PMID: 24826014]

[128] Basch, E.; Ulbricht, C.; Kuo, G.; Szapary, P.; Smith, M. Therapeutic applications of fenugreek. *Altern. Med. Rev.,* **2003**, *8*(1), 20-27.
[PMID: 12611558]

[129] Singh, P.; Singh, U.; Shukla, M.; Singh, R.L. Variation of some phytochemicals in methi and Saunf plants at different stages of development. *J Herb Med Toxicol,* **2010**, *4*(2), 93-99.

[130] Bukhari, S.B.; Bhanger, M.I.; Memon, S. Antioxidative activity of extracts from fenugreek seeds (*Trigonella foenum-graecum*). *Pak. J. Anal. Environ. Chem.,* **2008**, *9*(2), 78-83.

[131] Toppo, F.A.; Akhand, R.; Pathak, A.K. Pharmacological actions and potential uses of *Trigonella foenum-graecum*: A review. *Asian J. Pharm. Clin. Res.,* **2009**, *2*, 29-38.

[132] Singh, P.; Kakkar, P.; Singh, R.L. Protective effect of *Trigonella foecum graecum* and *Foeniculum vulgare* mature leaf against t-BHP induced toxicity in primary rat hepatocytes. *J. Excip. Food Chem.,* **2016**, *2*(111), 2472-0542.

[133] Tripathi, U.N.; Chandra, D. Hepatoprotective potential of Trigonella foenum graecum in deltamethrin induced albino rats. *Indian Journal of Pharmaceutical and Biological Research,* **2014**, *2*(4), 01-08.
[http://dx.doi.org/10.30750/ijpbr.2.4.1]

[134] Zargar, S. Protective effect of Trigonella foenum-graecum on thioacetamide induced hepatotoxicity in rats. *Saudi J. Biol. Sci.,* **2014**, *21*(2), 139-145.
[http://dx.doi.org/10.1016/j.sjbs.2013.09.002] [PMID: 24600306]

[135] Das, S. Hepatoprotective activity of methanolic extract of fenugreek seeds on rats. *Int. J. Pharm. Sci. Res.,* **2014**, *5*(4), 1506-1513.

[136] Tree, B. Aegle marmelos. available from:http://08hachi.blogspot.com/2011/08/aegle-marmelos.html

[137] Mohammad, A B N; Mannan, A; Nuruzzaman, M; Kamrujjaman, KM; Samir, K D Indigenous king of bitter (*Andrographis paniculata*): A review. *J. medicinal plants studies.,* **2017**, *5*(2), 318-324.

[138] How to plant and grow garlic in your veggie patch. available from: https://gardenerspath .com/plants/vegetables/growing-garlic/

[139] Remarkable benefits of onion (*allium cepa*). Available from:https://globalfoodbook.com/health-benefits-onion-allium-cepa

[140] Neem *Azadirachta Indica Ayur*. Available from:https://www.ayurtimes.com/neem-azadirachta-indica/

[141] Tabeshpour, J.; Imenshahidi, M.; Hosseinzadeh, H. A review of the effects of *Berberis vulgaris* and its major component, berberine, in metabolic syndrome. *Iran. J. Basic Med. Sci.,* **2017**, *20*(5), 557-568.
[PMID: 28656091]

[142] Boerhavia diffusa : Punarnava uses, benefits & dosage. Available from: https://www.planetayurveda .com/library/punarnava-boerhavia-diffusa/

[143] *Cassia fistula* – Iplantz. Available from:https://www.iplantz.com/plant/348/cassia-fistula/

[144] *Cissus quadrangularis* : Uses, benefits, side effects, and dosage. Available from:https://www. healthline.com/nutrition/cissus-quadrangularis

[145] Curcuma longa (*Curcumin*) dry extract : Panacea phytoextracts. Available from:https://www. panaceaphytoextracts.com/curcumin.php

[146] *Eclipta alba (Bhringraj)* benefits ,usage and dosage. Available from:https://www.planetayurveda .com/bhringraj-eclipta-alba/

[147] What are the health benefits of ginseng? Available from:https:// www.medicalnewstoday.com /articles/262982#_noHeaderPrefixedContent

[148] Indian biodiversity portal. Available from:https://indiabiodiversity.org/species/show/32210

[149] Holy basil (ocimum sanctum/ ocimum tenuiflorum). Available from:https://www.floralencounters .com/Seeds/seed_detail.jsp?grow=Basil+Holy&productid=1190

[150] Fruits of phyllanthus emblica l. - flickr - lalithamba. Available from:https://commons.wikimedia.org/ wiki/File:Fruits_of_Phyllanthus_emblica_L._-_Flickr_-_lalithamba.jpg

[151] Silymarin, a consistently amazing therapeutic agent. Available from:https://edu.emersonecologics .com/2017/09/11/silymarin-a-consistently-amazing-therapeutic-agent/

[152] available from: https://biodiversityofwestbengal.wildwingsindia.in/description.php?sname=Solanum% 20nigrum

[153] Arjuna (*Terminalia Arjuna*) properties ,benefits and usage. Available from:https://www.planeta-yurveda.com/library/arjuna-terminalia-arjuna/

[154] Ayush for immunity, guduchi (*Tinospora cordifolia*). Available from:https://morungexpress .com/ayush-for-immunity-guduchi-tinospora-cordifolia

[155] Encyclopedia britannica, fenugreek. Available from:https://www.britannica.com/plant/fenugreek

[156] Health benefits of Kutki. available from:https://www.healthbenefitstimes.com/kutki/

[157] Tejaswi, C; Abhijit, G; Manjiri, K Hepatoprotective activity of satwa, an ayurvedic formulation, against alcohol-induced liver injury in rats. *Altern Ther Health Med, 2017, 23*(4), 34-40.

[158] Vidhyotiny, B.; Udarrogchikitsa, Chaukhamba; Sanskrut, G.K.; Sansthan, Varanasi , 2004, 40, p. 432.

[159] Saraswat, B.; Visen, P.K.S.; Patnaik, G.K.; Dhawan, B.N. *Ex vivo* and *in vivo* investigations of picroliv from *Picrorhiza kurroa* in an alcohol intoxication model in rats. *J. Ethnopharmacol., 1999, 66*(3), 263-269.
[http://dx.doi.org/10.1016/S0378-8741(99)00007-0] [PMID: 10473171]

[160] Singh, S.S.; Pandey, S.C.; Srivastava, S.; Gupta, V.S.; Patro, B.; Ghosh, A.C. Chemistry and medicinal properties of *Tinospora cordifolia* (Guduchi). *Indian J. Pharm., 2003, 35*, 83-91.

[161] Ajith, T.A.; Hema, U.; Aswathy, M.S. Zingiber officinale Roscoe prevents acetaminophen-induced acute hepatotoxicity by enhancing hepatic antioxidant status. *Food Chem. Toxicol., 2007, 45*(11), 2267-2272.
[http://dx.doi.org/10.1016/j.fct.2007.06.001] [PMID: 17637489]

[162] Janbaz, K.H. Investigation of hepatoprotective activity of herbal constituents. phd thesis, department of pharmacology, faculty of pharmacy. University of Karachi, **1995**.

[163] Tasduq, S.A.; Singh, K.; Satti, N.K.; Gupta, D.K.; Suri, K.A.; Johri, R.K. *Terminalia chebula* (fruit) prevents liver toxicity caused by sub-chronic administration of rifampicin, isoniazid and pyrazinamide in combination. *Hum. Exp. Toxicol., 2006, 25*(3), 111-118.
[http://dx.doi.org/10.1191/0960327106ht601oa] [PMID: 16634329]

[164] Ghaisas, M.M.; Tanwar, M.B.; Ninave, P.B. Hepatoprotective activity of aqueous and ethanolic extract of *Trichosanthes dioica* Roxb. in ferrous sulphate-induced liver injury. *Pharmacologyonline,* **2008**, *3*, 127-135.

[165] Shah, V.N.; Shah, M.B.; Bhatt, P.A. Hepatoprotective activity of punarnavashtak kwath, an Ayurvedic formulation, against CCl4-induced hepatotoxicity in rats and on the HepG2 cell line. *Pharm. Biol.,* **2011**, *49*(4), 408-415.
[http://dx.doi.org/10.3109/13880209.2010.521162] [PMID: 21391842]

[166] Rohitakarista in bangladesh national formulary of ayurvedic medicine board of unani and ayurvedic system of medicine. Dhaka, Bangladesh, **1992**.

[167] Muhammad, N H; Ashik, M. Evaluation of hepatoprotective effect of a polyherbal formulation against carbon tetrachloride-induced hepatotoxicity in rats. *Altern Integr Med,* **2018**, *7*(2), 1-4.

[168] Tatiya, A.U.; Surana, S.J.; Sutar, M.P.; Gamit, N.H. Hepatoprotective effect of poly herbal

formulation against various hepatotoxic agents in rats. *Pharmacognosy Res.,* **2012**, *4*(1), 50-56.
[http://dx.doi.org/10.4103/0974-8490.91040] [PMID: 22224062]

[169] Gupta, A.; Sheth, N.R.; Pandey, S.; Shah, D.R.; Yadav, J.S. Design and evaluation of herbal hepatoprotective formulation against paracetamol induced liver toxicity. *J. Young Pharm.,* **2013**, *5*(4), 180-187.
[http://dx.doi.org/10.1016/j.jyp.2013.12.003] [PMID: 24563599]

[170] Tushar, K.B.; Kausik, C.; Debasis, D. Hepatoprotective activity of Livshis, a polyherbal formulation in CCl4-induced hepatotoxic male Wistar rats: A toxicity screening approachGenomic Medicine. *Biomarkers, and Health Sciences.,* **2011**, *3*(3-4), 103-110.

[171] Arsul, V.A.; Wagh, S.R.; Mayee, R. Hepatoprotective activity of livergen, a polyherbal formulation against carbon tetrachloride induced hepatotoxicity in rats. *Int. J. Pharm. Pharm. Sci.,* **2011**, *3*, 228-231.

[172] Bhattacharyya, D.; Pandit, S.; Mukherjee, R.; Das, N.; Sur, T.K. Hepatoprotective effect of Himoliv, a polyherbal formulation in rats. *Indian J. Physiol. Pharmacol.,* **2003**, *47*(4), 435-440.
[PMID: 15266956]

[173] Devaraj, V.C.; Krishna, B.G.; Viswanatha, G.L.; Kamath, J.V.; Kumar, S. Hepatoprotective activity of Hepax-a polyherbal formulation. *Asian Pac. J. Trop. Biomed.,* **2011**, *1*(2), 142-146.
[http://dx.doi.org/10.1016/S2221-1691(11)60013-0] [PMID: 23569745]

[174] Fiaz, M.; Fiaz, N.; Shakir, L.; Alamgeer, A.; Mehmood, W.; Mustafa, G.; Rauf, A.; Najam, K. Hepatoprotective effect of a polyherbal formulation and ascorbic acid in paracetamol induced hepatic damage in rabbits. *Biomed. Res. Ther.,* **2017**, *4*(4), 1261-1277.
[http://dx.doi.org/10.15419/bmrat.v4i4.161]

[175] Debendranath, D.; Sunetra, C.; Narendra, B.; Deepa, C. Hepatoprotective Activity of BV-7310, a Proprietary Herbal Formulation of *Phyllanthus niruri, Tephrosia purpurea, Boerhavia diffusa,* and *Andrographis paniculata,* in Alcohol Induced HepG2 Cells and Alcohol plusaHaloalkane,CCl4, Induced Liver Damage in Rats. *Evid. Based Complement. Alternat. Med.,* **2020**, •••, 1-9.

[176] Dandagi, P.M.; Patil, M.B.; Mastiholimath, V.S.; Gadad, A.P.; Dhumansure, R.H. Development and evaluation of hepatoprotective polyherbal formulation containing some indigenous medicinal plants. *Pharm. Sci.,* **2008**, *70*(2), 265-268.
[PMID: 20046731]

[177] Patere, S.N.; Saraf, M.N.; Majumdar, A.S. Hepatoprotective activity of polyherbal formulation (Normeta) in oxidative stress induced by alcohol, polyunsaturated fatty acids and iron in rats. *Basic Clin. Pharmacol. Toxicol.,* **2009**, *105*(3), 173-180.
[http://dx.doi.org/10.1111/j.1742-7843.2009.00418.x] [PMID: 19486336]

[178] Sivakumar, V.; Dhana, M.S.R.; Mohamed, A.; S Rajesh, K. Hepatoprotective effect of polyherbal formulations in paracetamol induced hepatic damaged experimental rat. *I. Res. J. Pharma.Biosci.,* **2014**, *1*(1), 30-35.

CHAPTER 5

Regulatory Affairs in Herbal Products

Megha Jha[1,*], Dolly Rani[2] and Kavita Chahal[3]

[1] *Department of Research, Pinnacle Biomedical Research Institute, Bhopal, M.P. 462003, India*

[2] *Amity Institutes of Pharmacy, Amity University, Noida-201303 India*

[3] *Department of Botany, Government College, Chhindwara, M.P. 480111, India*

Abstract: Various parameters/guidelines regulating the safety and efficacy of herbal pharmaceuticals, as well as their manufacturing and distribution, have been strongly implemented by regulatory bodies. To understand the pre-marketing requirements, the legislative status of herbal drugs/products was analyzed in this chapter for various countries in Southeast Asia, Africa, America, Europe, and Austria. Apart from the challenges of herb availability and conservation, it has been shown that there is a lack of harmony in the regulatory requirements for herbal products across the world. A critical evaluation was performed in order to detect the obstacles in the harmonization of herbal products. The worldwide trade and development of herbal products are being hampered by these issues. The herbal drug industry is inadequately regulated in most countries, and herbal medicines are often neither registered nor controlled. Quality compliance and assurance of the safety and efficacy of the marketed herbal drugs are major issues faced by developing as well as developed countries across the globe. The problem arises when herbal medication is utilized without legitimate permission, or in huge dosages, or in combination with other drugs for a longer period, or without discussion with a doctor, and produced properly. Taking these factors into account, the World Health Organization's International Drug Monitoring Program (WHO) has published standards for herbal assessment and quality control testing in order to improve the safety and efficacy of herbal-based therapeutics. This chapter covers the importance of regulatory affairs to be used in the processing of herbs and herbal products, and a comparative study of regulatory situations in different countries.

Keywords: Compliance, Harmonization, Legislative, Legitimate, Quality control, Regulatory affairs, Therapeutics.

1. INTRODUCTION

The World Health Organization's (WHO) International Drug Monitoring Program published certain recommendations for herbal drug evaluation and

* **Corresponding author Megha Jha:** Department of Research, Pinnacle Biomedical Research Institute, Bhopal, M.P. 462003, India; E-mail: meghajhabpl@gmail.com

Sachin Kumar Jain, Ram Kumar Sahu, Priyanka Soni, Vishal Soni & Shiv Shankar Shukla (Eds.)

quality control analysis. The World Health Organization has made a series of efforts to improve the safety and efficacy of herbal medicines. Toxicity from herbal medicines occurs if they're used without appropriate indications, in large doses, or in combination with other medications, for extended periods of time without seeking medical advice [1].

Regulatory affairs are initiated from government affairs that include controlling the safety and efficacy of herbal products in areas including pharmaceuticals, veterinary medicines, medical devices, pesticides, agrochemicals, cosmetics, and complementary medicines, for the protection of public health. It keeps track of the companies by establishing specialist departments of Regulatory Affairs professionals ensuring that they supply quality products to the public for their health and welfare. Because the production of herbal products takes time, from collection to manufacturing and packaging, Regulatory Affairs should be lead from the start to reduce the time required for the herbal product to reach the market, from developing effective regulatory strategies following the discovery of a new molecule to post-marketing planning, the Drug Regulatory Affairs (DRA) department or team a critical responsibility. Also, the cost-effective use of the company's resources has also increased by using regulatory affairs. Moreover, government authorities can easily rely upon scientifically knowledgeable company officials and hence, can work in cooperation with each other.

Scientists, regulators, industry, and, more recently, patient representatives and patient advocates have been brought together via research policies and alliances. In the near future, improved strategies for research-based corporate organizations, more integrated research tools dealing with appropriate translational requirements directed at clinical development, and proactive regulatory policies will be needed to accurately enhance the development of new technologies [2]. Depending on Ayurveda, a large no of companies are developing many products for therapeutic and supplementary uses. If we examine herbal products sold in India, we can easily find these don't bear product leaflet, which lacks usage instructions. When compared to allopathic medications, however, there is a significant difference. A pharmaceutical business invests a lot of money to prove its efficacy, which includes like bioavailability, toxicity, safety, clinical data, and so on. However, herbal products do not require this, and as a result, the majority of herbal products fail. If we look at the regulatory status of herbal products around the world, we can see how stringent other countries are when it comes to human safety [3].

The group of regulatory affairs is having a solid influential position that guarantees consistency with guidelines and empowers comprehension and understanding of a powerful regulation. Pharmaceutical, biologics, and medicine companies may be apprehensive if new products and processes are not thoroughly vetted and evaluated before they are published. However, failure to do so could result in the organization ceasing to evaluate marketing submissions in a timely and correct manner.

The key functions of the global regulatory affairs group include:

- Leading and providing strategic regulatory guidance and delivering the global regulatory strategy for product development, manufacturing, and registration.
- Building and maintaining a credible relationship with regulatory authorities with effective written and verbal communication.
- Establishing an efficient repository and archive for correspondence compliant with regulatory standards for audits.
- Providing high-quality, complete user/reviewer-friendly documents electronically transmissible and reproducible.
- Developing and maintaining product information and label.
- Providing regulatory intelligence, from paying attention to the regulatory environment and changing landscape, to participating in external industry partnerships and developing policy with regulatory agencies.
- Ensuring published information and promotional/advertising materials meet regulatory requirements.
- Ensuring functional units comply with regulatory requirements and good regulatory practices.

This end goal drives the need for the regulatory team to:

- Deliver innovative, breakthrough regulatory strategies for product development and registration.
- Become more anticipatory of the company's success imperatives.
- Be proactive and forward-thinking, and provide timely, comprehensive, and robust global regulatory guidance.
- Understand the biopharmaceutical environment and regulatory actions on precedents and utilize such regulatory intelligence.
- Forge new standards to deliver more predictable outcomes.

TRADITIONAL MEDICINE PROGRAMME BY WHO

The World Health Assembly (WHA) has posted numerous resolutions in recognition of this fact, and the Alma-Ata Declaration urges that scientific consensus on herbal medicines should be included in national drug policies and regulatory measures. As presented in the Forty-fourth World Health Assembly, it stated that "WHO collaborated with its Member States in the review of national policies, legislation and decisions on the nature and extent of the use of traditional medicine in their health systems." The major objectives set for Traditional Medicine Programme were to integrate traditional medicine into the national health care system, to set some technical guidelines and international standards for promoting herbal medicine, and to spread and promote various forms of traditional medicine.

The candor with which rich and developing countries alike assess their own traditional practices implies that progress is being made toward this goal. The current challenge is to improve the lines of action: evaluation, integration, and training. It is necessary to distinguish a myth from actuality in traditional doctors in order to discern authentic practices and remedies from those that are demonstrably ineffective and/or hazardous. As a consequence, WHO will continue to promote the development, teaching, and the use of analytical criteria for assessing the safety and efficacy of diverse parts of traditional medicine [4].

The Sixth International Conference on Drug Regulatory Authorities (ICDRA) in Ottawa, Canada, in October 1991, established Guidelines for the Assessment of Herbal Medicines as a consequence of a WHO consultation in Munich, Germany, in June 1991.

Regulations for the Formulation of National Policy on Herbal Medicines by the WHO Regional Office aimed to develop regulatory reforms to ensure health-care, ensuring the effectiveness of herbal medicines.

The major factors are:

1. Recognizing ancient medicine as a vital component of the healthcare system.

2. Establishing a partnership between traditional and contemporary medicine.

3. Advancing the utilization of items in a sensible manner.

4. Putting in place quality assurance methods.

5. Assuring that supplies would be available on a regular basis.

6. Advancing regulatory measure research and development.

7. A reliable supply of medicinal plants, including collection, cultivation, local manufacture and processing, imports, and stora ge.

8. Establishing rules and regulations to ensure those plants and their products are of high quality.

9. Identifying and assuring the safety and efficacy of herbal medicines for direct

use in national healthcare systems.

10. Developing criteria and broad concepts to guide research on herbal medicines evaluation.

11. Advancing their rational application.

12. Establishing research criteria for their assessment.

13. Overcoming legal stumbling blocks to herbal medication use.

14. Taking into account traditional preparation experience, encompassing long-term use, as well as medical and ethnological background

15. Facilitating the proper use of herbal medicines by developing a technical guide for basic health care called "WHO Monographs on Selected Medicinal Plants."

16. Part I covers each plant's botanical properties, active chemical ingredients, and quality control; Part II covers clinical uses, pharmacology, posology, potential contraindications, and precautions.

FACTORS USED IN HERBAL MEDICINAL PRODUCT CLASSIFICATION IN REGULATORY SYSTEMS

• Description in Pharmacopoeia monograph.
• Ingredients or substances that are listed on a schedule and that are regulated.
• Claim of a therapeutic effect.
• Prescription status.
• Period of use.

INTERNATIONAL REGULATORY LEGISLATIONS

Different countries have their own different legislations regarding herbal preparations and products. Some jurisdictions have formally recognized herbal medications, while others have a unique licensing system in place to allow health authorities to test ingredients and quality to guarantee that they are used properly and safely before they are promoted.

GLOBAL MARKET

The global market is divided into two categories as Fig. (**1**) shows.

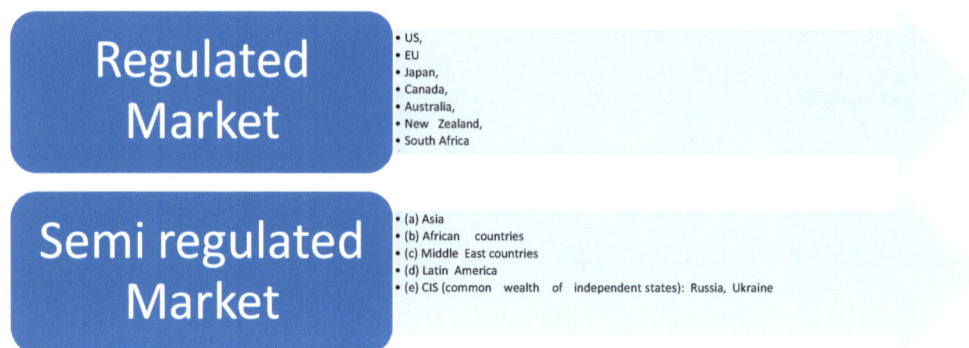

Regulated Market
- US,
- EU
- Japan,
- Canada,
- Australia,
- New Zealand,
- South Africa

Semi regulated Market
- (a) Asia
- (b) African countries
- (c) Middle East countries
- (d) Latin America
- (e) CIS (common wealth of independent states): Russia, Ukraine

Fig. (1). Categories of Global Market.

South Africa

Traditional healers are the primary doctors for a huge majority of South Africans. In the country, there are over 200,000 traditional healers, and the trading of native herbal products is largely unregulated. However, once a health-related claim is put on a finished product, the drug control committee must approve it before it may be marketed. New "traditional" herbal remedies are not subject to any special registration or regulatory procedures. Ancient remedies, such as senna leaf or aloe vera, have been registered with the MCC in accordance with internationally recognized standards of efficacy and safety.

The United States Pharmacopeia (USP) or the British Pharmacopeia (BP) should be used as a guideline for pharmaceutical standards [5].

MCC traditional herbs laws are similar to FDA standards previous to the Dietary Supplement Health and Education Act of 1994. As a part of government reconstruction and development plan, traditional medicine is incorporated into the medical policy. The Traditional Medicine Project (TRAMED) of the University of Cape Town's, Department of Pharmacology was involved in planning for the registration and control of Traditional medicines in 1994. The major goals of this project were to promote safe, effective, high-quality "essential" traditional medicines, as well as scientific verification and primary healthcare, by providing therapists with important information and training [6].

The Americas

Canada

Herbal medicines or drugs must comply with the labeling and other requirements stipulated in the Food and Drug Act and regulations. So, as compared to the United States, a large number of prescription herbal medications are legal in Canada Market. Before assigning a registration number or drug identification number, it is necessary to carefully check the composition and the label of the drug. On August 13, 1987, after a lengthy discussion between stakeholders and experts, the Canadian Health Protection Agency issued an information letter containing a list of herbal medications that were deemed dangerous or required attention on labelling.

Since January 2004, Health Canada has governed herbal remedies and traditional medicines notably Ayurvedic medicine under the Natural Health Products Regulations. A manufacturer, packer, labeller, or importer must first be registered with Health Canada before commencing any such activity, according to the regulations.

The process includes registering the manufacturing facility as well as the products. The Natural Health Product Directorate requires complete data on product composition, standardization, stability, microbial and chemical contaminant testing methods and tolerance limits, safety and efficacy, constituent characterization, and quantification by assay or by input (NHPD).NHPs must satisfy contaminant limitations and be manufactured according to GMP guidelines, according to the authorities [7].

The pharmacological activity of the component, as well as the product's use and declaration of use, decide whether an herbal product is a food or a medication.In 1992, the HPB presented a regulatory proposal to the Canadian Parliament that included a list of 64 more plants that were designated adulterants. The Canadian regulatory system is in conformity with WHO criteria for herbal medication evaluation [8, 9].

Clinical studies on human subjects are also suggested for finding or verifying the product's effects, detecting any adverse events associated with its usage, investigating its absorption, distribution, metabolism, and excretion, and evaluating its safety or efficacy [10].

United States of America

Herbal products are not very popular in the United States. As it is only accessible in health food stores, which are only visited by a small percentage of the population, this is the case. Because medical claims cannot be submitted and consumers rely on pharmacists' advice, expanding distribution through pharmacies is challenging. They usually have minimal knowledge about herbal medicine.

The Food, Drugs, and Cosmetics Act was passed in the late 1930s. Since then, any items intended to treat, cure, alleviate, or prevent diseases have been regulated as medicines by the (FDA). As a result, the same procedures as for chemical drugs must be followed to authorize any herbal claims. Most natural items are classified as food or food additives in the United States, despite the fact that consumers use them as folk medicine. As a result, the majority of regulatory activities are focused on security.

When herbal remedy is classified as "generally recognized as safe" (GRAS), it signifies that no claims have been made and the product has not been mislabelled or contaminated. Natural products can possibly be classified as GRAS if certified specialists affirm it and no other experts disagree.

The FDA lists some well-known herbal treatments as over-the-counter pharmaceuticals. However, most of these herbs have been rejected as a result of an 18-year evaluation of over-the-counter pharmaceuticals, mostly because the US herbal business has not given data to justify their usage. The FDA formed a new non-prescription drug external expert advisory group in November 1992 [11].

Herbal medicines are not drugs, according to civil legislation governing the health food industry. This rule bans the FDA from issuing monographs for dietary supplements, vitamins, minerals, and herbal medicines in the same way that it does for other pharmaceuticals. The government approved the Nutrition Labelling and Education Act (NLEA) in 1990, requiring all foods to carry nutrition labels and for the FDA to set guidelines for approving food health benefits.

Dietary supplements have been proved to reduce chronic disease and hence assist decrease the expenses of long-term medicals, according to the Dietary Supplements Health and Education Act [12] passed in 1994. Dietary supplements currently include herbs and other botanicals, vitamins, and minerals. They are available as tablets and liquids.

Dietary supplements do not include chemicals that were initially marketed as pharmaceuticals and afterward marketed as dietary supplements, nor substances that have undergone clinical research but were not first marketed as dietary supplements [12].

Eastern Mediterranean

Saudi Arabia

According to Article 44 and Article 50 of the "Pharmaceutical Industry and Pharmaceutical TradeAct"promulgated by Royal Decree No. M/18 on March 18, 1398, the registration of medicines by the Ministry of Health is mandatory. Section 13A of the RegistrationRegulations amended by Ministerial Resolution 06/17/1409 No. 1214/20 specifically requires registration, except for medicines, products with medicinal effects, or products containing active ingredients with medicinal effects, such as herbal preparations, Health and supplementary foods, medicinal, preservatives or medical devices.

Herbal products are classified in Saudi Arabia as traditional products. They are permitted if they were used for at least 50 years in a row. Their quantity and preparation procedure must be the same as those used in the past.

According to the evidence provided, they may fall under the sub-categories:

- Pharmacopoeia evidence for traditional products
- Nonpharmacopoeial evidence for traditional products.

The medicinal ingredients, quantity, recommended dose, route of administration, duration of use, dosage form, directions of use, and risk information for the former should be identical to those in the Pharmacopeia, and the methodology of preparation must be customary [13].

Herbal preparations are defined as products for therapeutic and/or preventive purposes, the active ingredients of which are derived from plants. This definition is limited to preparations for topical, oral, rectal, or inhalation administration. World Health Organization/TRM/98.1 has "Saudi Arabia" under the "Regulations on the Registration of Herbal Preparations, Health and Supplementary Foods, and Preservatives". As a result, information on ingredients, treatment categories, certificates of analysis, and alcohol percentages must be included in papers such as manufacture licenses, free sales certificates, and GMP certificates, as well as the type of animal (if it is of animal origin).

Europe

In general, the European Community has established a comprehensive legal framework to facilitate the free movement of products, capital, services, and people inside the EU. Medicines must get pre-market authorization under Directives 65/65 / EEC and 75/318 / EEC before they can be sold.

The 91/507/EEC [14] Official Journal of the European Communities nE L. 270/32 of 26 September 1991.] The directive specifies requirements for quality, safety, and effective documents, files, and expert reports. 75/319/EEC [15].

Austria

Drugs made from chemicals and those made from plants are not differentiated in Austrian legislation. Certain over-the-counter drugs may have their registration fees lowered. Article 17a of the Austrian Drug Law [16] mentions this. This means that there isn't a thorough assessment of quality and safety. The following is a list of active ingredients and excipients that comply with the simplified procedure that was published in 1989 [17]and was last revised in 1992 [18].

Make a list of roughly 500 medical substances and plants/plant parts/essential oils, and so on. It is possible to apply the simpler technique described in section 17a. Sections 15 and 17 of the Austrian Drug Law list the mandatory paperwork requirements. Pharmacies are the only places where pharmaceuticals can be purchased. Article 59.3 of the Austrian Medicines Act establishes an exemption, allowing some products to be sold outside pharmacies, such as in pharmacies, without posing any risk. Officially published is a list of these goods, many of which are medical plants, with descriptions of medicinal plants/sections of plants, indications, and dose recommendations.

Germany

Herbal medicine accounts for a sizable portion of the German pharmaceutical sector. According to a report presented at the ESCOP meeting in Brussels in October 1990 [19]. ESCOP, 1990., the German herbal medicine market was valued at US $ 1.7 billion in 1989 (including the tax on value-added), accounting for 10% of the overall German pharmaceutical market.

In June 1989, the Allensbach Institute [20] conducted representative research in a German community, which confirmed that a considerable proportion of people utilize natural remedies. Herbal medication is totally considered medicine in terms of legal position. In 1992, the Court of Justice of the European Communities reaffirmed this legal stance.

Certification of quality, safety, and efficacy became a requirement for drug registration under this new legislation. Member states are required by the Council Directive 75/319 / EEC.

Article 39, paragraph 2, assessed all products on the market at the time within 12 years to establish if they are compliant with European directives.

During the 12-year transition period, that is, until December 31, 1989 (and subsequently extended to April 30, 1990) these products were allowed to continue to be sold under the so-called "fiction marketing authorization". Authorities were required to perform a review procedure in order to comply with the criteria of the new "Drug Law". Existing product evaluation is a two-step procedure. When the Drug Law was updated for the fifth time in 1994, it was largely discontinued. The technique is divided into two steps: the first is a review of the active substances that results in a monograph, and the second is the specific verification of the drug [21].

United Kingdom

The conditions for the UK licensing system are laid forth in Part II of the Medicines Act 1968. It is illegal to manufacture, sell, provide, export, or import medications in the United Kingdom without the required licenses unless certain exemptions or rules apply.

Article 12 of the Pharmaceutical Law provides for the license exemption for certain herbal medicines, namely: Plants only undergo drying, crushing, or crushing process during the production of herbal medicines; They are sold or provided under their botanical names in connection to the manufacturing method; - sold or supplied without any explicit treatment advice.

Herbs used under self-diagnosing conditions are approved after establishing sufficient evidence of efficacy. Authorities require that product labels include "medicinal herbs traditionally used to relieve symptoms of ..." and "If symptoms persist, consult your doctor."Combination products with a significant number of herbal compounds or a mixture of herbal and non-herbal ingredients are not acceptable, and licensees are asked to think about which ingredients the treatment claims refer to and adapt the recipe accordingly [22].

South East Asia

India

Herbal medicines are regulated under the Rules 1945 and 1940 Drug and Cosmetic Act (D and C) based on regulatory provisions for Ayurveda, Unani, Siddha medicine. AYUSH is the regulatory authority and implements that herbal drug manufacturing will be done after getting a manufacturing license, as applicable.

- The D and C Act covers licensing, composition, manufacture, labeling, packing, quality, and export. Schedule "T" of the act lays down the good manufacturing practice (GMP). The first schedule of the D and C Act have to be followed for licensing any herbal product under the two broad areas:
- ASU drugs
- Patent or proprietary medicines [23]

Ordinary Indians are well-versed in the ancient applications of plants. Because most practitioners formulate and distribute their own prescriptions, it's difficult to estimate the market size of the traditional Indian system. The yearly turnover of large-scale items is expected to be around $300 million, while the turnover of modern pharmaceuticals is estimated to be around $2.5 billion.

Despite certain prescriptions, general practitioners are unfamiliar with Ayurvedic remedies, according to a study on the attitudes of modern medical professionals regarding Ayurvedic items. They are willing to test Ayurvedic products if their efficacy has been scientifically demonstrated, and if no contemporary medical treatment is available, they will attempt Ayurvedic products. Self-medication is used to treat mild illnesses.

Ayurvedic remedies are available in pharmacies without a prescription. These items appear to be an essential part of the Indian brands' traditional offerings. To be legitimate and acceptable to all, Ayurveda still needs empirical support from modern medical research. Traditional medical systems' benefits in terms of safety and efficacy are being defined through innovative research activities [24].

In India, the Ayurvedic system currently has approximately 250,000 registered practitioners (total of all traditional systems: approximately 291,000), while the modern medical system has approximately 700,000. In all states of India, conventional system doctors comprise about one-third of government medical employment.

Traditional medicines in India are supervised by the Medicines and Cosmetics Act of 1940 and the Medicines and Cosmetics Regulations of 1945. Medicines and cosmetics are regulated in terms of import, manufacture, distribution, and sale. The Indian government acknowledged traditional Indian medicine in 1959, and the Drugs and Cosmetics Act was changed to cover medicines derived from Indian traditional medicine.Without the authorization of the national drug control authority, the manufacture of items derived from traditional systems is prohibited. Patents and patented medicines derived from traditional systems must contain the components listed in the acknowledged books of the aforementioned systems, according to the regulations of the "Law on Medicines and Cosmetics."

The government receives guidance from special committees and advisory committees for Ayurveda, Siddha, and Unani medicines. To produce a pharmacopeia for all of these systems, a pharmacopeia committee was formed [25].

In 1993, the Government of India formed an expert committee to produce standards for the safety and efficacy of herbal medicines with the goal of adding them to the Drugs and Cosmetics Act and standards.

Only herbs allowed by the licensor, as well as plants mentioned and produced according to the formulas in the "authorization" books of Ayurveda, Siddha, and Unani herbs, must be developed or sold. Manufacturers of experimental herbal medicines must provide sufficient safety and efficacy proof in their marketing authorization applications.

It is suggested that herbal medications be classified according to their market availability and their nature:

-Category 1: Drugs that have been in use for more than 5 years

-Category 2: Drugs that have been in use for less than 5 years

-Category 3: New drugs Herbs are classified according to whether they contain processed or unprocessed plant parts, as well as whether or not they contain potentially dangerous plants.

Product classification and market availability influence the safety and efficacy criteria. Clinical trial data and toxicity data submission criteria vary depending on the type of herbal medicine and the market supply [26].

AYUSH department, ICMR and CSIR jointly work to achieve the goal of safe and effectual AYUSH products for various therapeutic diseases and for manufacturing of novel drugs in India. Herbal drugs come under Drug and Cosmetics act 1940, and Rules 1945(D & C ACT). As per rule, Ayurvedic, Unani or Siddha drugs include all medicines for internal and external use or used in the diagnosis of disease, treatment of disease, mitigation or curing the disease or disorder in human beings or animals, and manufactured completely according the formulae described in the valid books of Siddha, the system of Ayurvedic and Unani medicine, given in the very First Schedule. The D&C Act extends the control over licensing, formulation composition, manufacture, labelling, packing, quality, and export. Schedule "T" of the act gives us Good Manufacturing Practice (GMP) requirements that is carried for the manufacture of herbal drugs.

The main objective is to upgrade the educational standards of Indian System in Medicines and Homoeopathy Universities and college in the country. Their main objective is to control drug quality, laying down pharmacopeial standards, overseeing working of pharmacopeial Laboratory of Indian Medicines, by the Quality Council of India and observing the process of Indian Medicine Pharmaceutical Company Limited. AYUSH also controls implementation of Good Manufacturing Practices, setting up of common facilities following Cluster approach and executing the scheme on Drug Quality Control with the disclosure of herbal medical formulations, knowledge & manuscripts, documentation and promotion of regional health traditions. AYUSH department together with Quality Council of India established a certification scheme for AYUSH drug products. Always people were concerned for the standards of AYUSH products with regard to their quality, safety and efficacy. To satisfy these concerns, a new scheme of voluntary certification of AYUSH products has been started with the Quality Council of India [27, 28].

Malaysia

In Malaysia, herbal drugs are categorized as regulating products. Any herbal product seller needs to register the herbal product before selling it. They need to file an application to the Malaysia Registrar of Business or Suruhanjaya Syarikat Malaysia under two classifications:

- Traditional products
- Health supplements

While the authorities demand the phrase "traditionally used for" to appear in front of any claim made on a traditional product, only those functional claims specified by the authority are permitted in supplements [29].

Traditional Chinese Medicine

In terms of their legal backing, Chinese herbal medicines are generally represented as medications that require additional documentation, such as quality files, safety and effectiveness studies, and unique labels, in order to be commercialized. New drugs must be tested and approved in accordance with the "Drug Administration Law". After approval, the new drug certificate will receive the approval number. Then allow the factory to sell the product.This process respects traditional knowledge while evaluating the efficacy and quality of enhanced traditional medicines and administratively contributing to the growth of traditional medicine.

On September 20, 1984, the People's Republic of China passed the Drug Administration Law."The state fosters the development of contemporary and traditional medicines, which play an essential role in disease prevention and treatment," says Article 3. The state protects wild medicinal resources and encourages the cultivation of domestic medicinal materials. ", Article 5 stipulates that"they must be equipped with a sufficient number of pharmacists or technicians with the title of an associate engineer or higher and qualified workers suitable for the scale of pharmaceutical production.

Article 6 stipulates that "the processing of medicinal plant materials must be prepared and cut in accordance with the provisions of the Pharmacopoeia of the People's Republic of China or the processing specifications prescribed by the health bureau of the province, autonomous region or municipality directly under the Central Government". With regard to the control of commercial pharmaceutical companies, Article 11 stipulates that commercial pharmaceutical companies must be equipped with a sufficient number of pharmacy technicians equal with the commercial scale. However, in the absence of pharmaceutical technicians, modern pharmaceutical companies may employ pharmaceutical professionals who are familiar with the nature of drugs and are registered with the health office at or above the county level. Article 15 stipulates that, with certain exceptions, the sale of medicinal plant materials is only allowed in the rural market. Article 29 stipulates that "if the domestic market for medicinal plant materials and patented herbal medicines are scarce, the Ministry of Health has the right to restrict or prohibit exports." Article 31 stipulates that "without the approval of the health department of a province, autonomous region, or municipality directly under the Central Government, no newly discovered or imported medicinal plant materials may be sold abroad" [30].

New traditional Chinese medicine preparations; - TCM mixed preparations with TCM as the principal element; - historically imported growing materials make up the third category. The fourth category includes innovative traditional Chinese medicine formulations or administration routes, as well as materials imported from other parts of the country and materials cultivated rather than collected in nature. In clinical research requirements, medicinal materials report must include the following elements: research purpose, previous experience or modern research data, source of materials, cultivation, processing, properties, pharmacological and empirical data, toxicity data (only applies to category 1), draught quality standards, stability, and clinical research proposal plans. Quality standards, stability testing, clinical research abstracts, and packaging materials must all be included in a separate production application. Depending on the drug category, the pharmaceutical preparation report should meet the same requirements as the medicinal material report. In a separate paragraph, the technological prerequisites for pharmacological research are outlined.The uniqueness of traditional Chinese medicines should be taken into account while designing the main efficacy trials. The effects of the primary medications should be studied using two or more ways, depending on the new drug's influence on the syndrome or condition. This investigation should be sufficient to verify the major therapeutic functions and additional important therapeutic functions of the first, second, and third novel medications [31].

Rules, Laws and Governing Body

In India, the Drug and Cosmetic Act 1940 and Drug and Cosmetic Rule, which were modified in numerous states, were the first to provide a national policy on complementary and alternative medicine. The Indian government revised the Drug and Cosmetic Act in 1959 and acknowledged the traditional Indian System of Medicine (ISM). A number of expert committees for various ISMs were periodically constituted, with the first one being created in 1962. Act 13 of 1964 added a second chapter to the Act in 1969 that dealt with Ayurveda, Siddha, and Unani medicines. This chapter was partially identical to those for conventional pharmaceuticals. Later, in the years 1983, 1987, 1994, and 2002, the act underwent another change with a few substitutions.

The Central Council of Indian Medicine (CCIM) was established in 1970 and has since been active in establishing and enforcing a number of rules, including those governing ISM curricula and syllabi (*i.e.* Ayurveda, Siddha, and Unani). The CCIM includes the Sowa Rigpa medical system as of 2012. With the intention of developing the ISM, the Department of Indian Medicine and Homeopathy (ISM & H) was established. This department was renamed the Department of Ayurveda, Yoga, Naturopathy, Unani, Siddha, and Homoeopathy (AYUSH) in 2003, and a new ministry for AYUSH was established in 2014. Only after receiving IEC and DCG's written consent may a clinical trial be started. Applications are submitted using form 44 and must be accompanied by the requirements listed in Table **1** of Schedule Y, which may include documentation including information on chemicals, pharmaceuticals, animal pharmacology, toxicology, and clinical pharmacology data [32].

Table. 1 Supporting Documentation for Clinical trails.

Form of D and C Act	
Form 44	Application to take clinical trial, import and manufacturing permission.
Form 12	Application for licence to import drugs for the purpose of analysis.
Form 11	License to import drugs for analysis.

(Table 1) cont.....

Form of D and C Act	
Form 44	Import certificate issuance.
Form 1	Application form for issue certificate for import of narcotics.
Rule 34	Request for license for test and analysis.
Rule 122-A	Application for permission to import new drug
Rule 122-DA	Application for permission to conduct clinical trials for drug development
Rule 55	Application for import certificate
Rule 56	Issue of import certificate

CONCLUSION

Globally, consumers are increasingly accepting herbal products used in health care, beauty, and dietary supplements. For economic reasons, researchers and the pharmaceutical industry are paying more and more attention to the herbal industry. Herbal products are allowed to be traded legally. These products show growth opportunities for herbal products in their country. However, due to different regulatory requirements related to quality, safety, and efficacy data, there are differences in the status of ingredients and excipients, and challenges such as developing globally acceptable products are hindering the development of food industry. The global harmonization of herbal product regulations will work towards providing the much-needed impetus to this potential market segment.

LIST OF ABBREVIATIONS

TRAMED	Traditional Medicine Project
GMP	Good manufacturing practice
I.D.M.P.	International Drug Monitoring Program
DRA	Drug Regulatory Affairs
WHA	World Health Assembly
ICDRA	International Conference on Drug Regulatory Authorities
NHPD	Natural Health Product Directorate
ESCOP	European Scientific Cooperative on Phytotherapy
TCM	Traditional Chinese medicine

REFERENCES

[1]   Hooda, R.; Pandita, D.; Kumari, P.; Lather, V. Regulatory and quality aspects of herbal drugs. *Appl. Clin. Res. Clin. Trials Regul. Aff.,* **2017**, *4*(2), 107-113.
[http://dx.doi.org/10.2174/2213476X046661706190922022]

[2]   Sainz, V.; Conniot, J.; Matos, A.I.; Peres, C.; Zupančič, E.; Moura, L.; Silva, L.C.; Florindo, H.F.; Gaspar, R.S. Regulatory aspects on nanomedicines. *Biochem. Biophys. Res. Commun.,* **2015**, *468*(3),

504-510.
[http://dx.doi.org/10.1016/j.bbrc.2015.08.023] [PMID: 26260323]

[3]   Giri, RP; Gangawane, AK; Giri, SG Regulation on herbal product used as medicine around the world:
        A review. *IRJET,* **2018**, *5*(10)

[4]   Akerele, O. WHO's traditional medicine programme: Progress and perspectives. *WHO Chron.,* **1984**,
        38(2), 76-81.
        [PMID: 6475036]

[5]   Gericke, N. The regulation and control of traditional herbal medicines. **1995**. Available
        from:http://apps. who. int/medicinedocs/pdf/whozip57e/whozip57e. pdf (Accessed-December 2011)

[6]   Felhaber, T.; Gericke, N.T. Final narrative report: 1 June 1994-30 April 1996. *Traditional Medicines
        Programme at the University of Cape Town,* **1996**.

[7]   Health Canada. Natural Health Products – Drugs and Health Products: Ottawa, **2013**.

[8]   Zhang, X. Regulatory situation of herbal medicines : A worldwide review. In: *Traditional Medicine
        Programme*; World Health Organization., **1998**.

[9]   Adhami, H.R.; Mesgarpour, B.; Farsam, H. Herbal medicine in iran. *HerbalGram,* **2007**, *74*, 35-43.

[10]   o'Sullivan, T. Report on the regulation of complementary and alternative practitioners in Ireland.

[11]   Kuipers, S.E.; Farnsworth, N.R.; Fong, H.M.; Segelman, A.B. Herbal medicines-a continuing world
        trend. *1st World Federation of Proprietary Medicine Manufacturers Asia Pacific Regional Meeting,*
        Jakarta

[12]   Congress, U.S. **1994**.The dietary supplement health and education act of 1994: public law 103-417.
        103rd Congress of the United States of America,

[13]   Saudi food and drug authority. kingdom of saudi arabia: data requirements for herbal and health
        products submission: contents of dossier, version 1. **2012**.

[14]   Commission directive 91/507/eec of 19 july 1991 modifying the annex to council directive 75/318/eec
        on the approximation of the laws of member states relating to analytical, pharmacotoxicological and
        clinical standards and protocols in respect of the testing of medicinal products. *Official Journal of the
        European Communities nE L. 270/32,* **1991**.

[15]   Council Directive 75/319/EEC of 20 May 1975 on the approximation of provisions laid down by law,
        regulation or administrative action relating to proprietary medicinal products. *Official Journal of the
        European Communities nE L 147,* **1975**.

[16]   Medicines Act. Federal Law Gazette for the Republic of Austria No. 185/1983, amended by Federal
        Laws BGBl. No. 748/1988, No. 45/1991 and .../1993. **1993**.

[17]   Ordinance of the federal minister for health and public service of october 16, 1989 regarding
        simplifications in the approval of certain medicinal products. federal law gazette for the republic of
        austria 1989:3641-3666. **1989**.

[18]   Ordinance of the federal minister for health, sport and consumer protection, which amends the
        ordinance regarding simplifications in the approval of certain medicinal products. In: *Federal Law
        Gazette for the Republic of Austria*; , **1992**; pp. 3912-3915.

[19]   Bieldermann, B.J. Phytopharmaceuticals-The growing European market. *In Presentation at the
        ESCOP Symposium European harmony in phytotherapy,* **1990**, *20*

[20]   Berichte, A. The young generation turns to natural remedies Zur. *Bundestag printed matter,* **1989**, *11*,
        2915.

[21]   Keller, K. Results of the revision of herbal drugs in the federal republic of germany with a special
        focus on risk aspects. *Z. Phytother.,* **1992**, *13*, 116-120.

[22]   The Medicines Act, London HMSO. **1968**.

[23]   India, Malik V. Law relating to drugs and cosmetics: Containing drugs & cosmetics act, 1940, drugs and cosmetics rules, 1945 along with drugs (prices control) order, 2013, national pharmaceuticals pricing policy, 2012 (nppp-2012), pharmacy act, 1948, poisons act, 1919, drugs and magic remedies (objectionable advertisements) act, 1954 and other allied acts, rules etc. with information on herbal formulations, cosmetics and extracts, etc. eastern book company, **2014**.

[24]   Rajagopalan, T.G. Traditional herbal medicines around the globe: modern perspectives. *The Indian Perspective Proceedings of the 10th General Assembly of WFPMM, Seoul, Korea. Swiss Pharma.,* **1991**, *13*(11a), pp. 63-67.

[25]   Chakravarty, B.K. Herbal medicines. safety and efficacy guidelines. *Regul. Aff. J.,* **1993**, *4*, 699-701.

[26]   Kumar, V. Herbal medicines: Overview on regulations in india and south africa. *World J. Pharm. Res.,* **2017**, *6*(8), 690-698.
       [http://dx.doi.org/10.20959/wjpr20178-9091]

[27]   Sharma, S. Current status of herbal product: Regulatory overview. *J. Pharm. Bioallied Sci.,* **2015**, *7*(4), 293-296.
       [http://dx.doi.org/10.4103/0975-7406.168030] [PMID: 26681886]

[28]   Ishak, R.; Mohamad, J. Guidelines on registration of traditional and health supplement products. In: *Revised ed. Version 1.0*; Malaysian Biotechnology Corporation SDN BH: Kuala Lumpur, **2011**.

[29]   Drug administration law of the people's republic of china. , **1984**.

[30]   Mangathayaru, K. Pharmacognosy: An indian perspective. Pearson, **2013**.

[31]   Anonymous amendments and notifications drugs and cosmetics rules. **1945**.

[32]   World health organization. WHO; Geneva:National policy on traditional medicine and regulation of herbal medicines. *Report of a WHO Global Survey,* **2005**.

CHAPTER 6

Hepatoprotective Effects of Edible Plants and Spices

Raja Chakraborty[1,*] and **Saikat Sen**[2]

[1] *Institute of Pharmacy, Assam Don Bosco University, Tapesia Gardens, Sonapur – 782 402, Assam - India*

[2] *Faculty of Pharmaceutical Science, Assam down town University, Guwahati, Assam, India*

Abstract: Liver diseases are considered a major global public health problem that is always underestimated. Damage to hepatocytes caused by drugs, toxins, viruses, *etc.* is a major cause of hepatic disorders, including liver cancer. Oxidative stress is considered a primary underlying mechanism of liver disorders. Cytokine produced in response to ROS plays an important role in damaging the liver. Plants are also considered an important source of phytoconstituents with hepatoprotective activity. As part of the diet, edible plants could play an important role in protecting the liver from injury caused by oxidative stress, microorganisms, or other exogenous substances. Many vegetables, fruits, and spices have been investigated for their hepatoprotective activity in pre-clinical studies. Phytoconstituents like curcumin, catechin, rutin, myristicin, fumaric acid, silybin, picroside, kutkoside, glycyrrhizin, silymarin, and apigenin were found to exhibit hepatoprotective and antioxidant activity through diverse mechanisms including antioxidant activity, and anti-inflammatory activity. This chapter highlighted edible plants with hepatoprotective activity.

Keywords: Antioxidant, Edible plant, Hepatoprotective activity, Phytochemicals.

INTRODUCTION

The liver is the largest organ of the human body that plays a central role in the metabolism of exogenous substances and eliminating toxins. The liver consists of almost 2–5% of the adult body weight and approximately 10% of the blood flowing through the liver [1, 2]. The liver also assists in converting essential micronutrients into usable forms required by the human body and accomplishes more than 500 different functions. Damage to hepatic cells is a significant problem and is responsible for a broad spectrum of liver diseases. Endogenous

* **Corresponding author Raja Chakraborty:** Institute of Pharmacy, Assam Don Bosco University, Tapesia Gardens, Sonapur – 782 402, Assam - India; Tel: 7002171166; E-mail: dr_rchakraborty@rediffmail.com

Sachin Kumar Jain, Ram Kumar Sahu, Priyanka Soni, Vishal Soni & Shiv Shankar Shukla (Eds.)

substances like drugs, toxins, viruses, *etc* are a major cause of hepatic disorders [1].

Different liver diseases are considered a major global public health problem that is always underestimated. A global survey almost eight years ago estimated that 844 million people suffer from chronic liver diseases (CLDs), with more than 2 million deaths/year. Complications of cirrhosis, viral hepatitis and hepatocellular carcinoma are considered a major cause of death associated with liver diseases. A recent rise in the number of non-alcoholic steatohepatitis (NASH) was also reported [3, 4]. Alcohol-associated liver disease (AALD) is considered the main reason for liver disease. Alcohol usually causes liver injury and coexists with viral hepatitis and other infections. While non-alcoholic fatty liver diseases like non-alcoholic fatty liver (*i.e.* steatosis or steatosis) and NASH (*i.e* fibrosis, cirrhosis, carcinoma) are also responsible for wide range of complications [4]. Hepatocellular carcinoma (HCC) is the most frequent primary liver malignancy associated with a large number of deaths and is considered the foremost reason for global cancer-related death. CLDs and liver cirrhosis continue as leading reasons for the development of HCC. Many factors like viral hepatitis and excessive alcohol intake are considered major underlying causes associated with such conditions [5]. The consumption of excessive alcohol is associated with a spectrum of liver injury. Excessive alcohol intake enhances NADH levels that alter the cellular redox potential and increase the synthesis of lipids. Alcohol consumption is also associated with enhanced generation of free radicals and increases the expression of lipogenic enzymes and cytokines. Sterol regulatory element binding protein-1c (SREBP-1c) and early growth response-1 (Egr-1) are linked and play an important role in such conditions. Regular and excessive intake of alcohol results in different hepatic lesions associated with steatosis, fibrosis, hepatitis, and cirrhosis. Inflammation, destruction of parenchyma, and free radical generation lead to fibrosis and cirrhosis [6]. Viral hepatitis is closely linked with the pathogenesis of chronic liver disease. It was estimated that approximately 400 million people are affected by either hepatitis B and C infection [2].

Good food always boosts health, and bioactive components present in the food always play a vital role in preserving and maintaining health. Through diet, we receive an adequate amount of nutrients, antioxidants, and other bioactive molecules that are in synergy, and promote health. Bioactive molecules present in food besides the protein, fat, carbohydrates, vitamins, and minerals play an important role in maintaining health [7]. Oxidative stress is considered a situation caused by the increase in the generation of ROS/RNS or depletion of antioxidant defence. ROS may cause major damage to the liver. Parenchymal cells are the principal target of ROS and linked with liver injury. Cytokines produced in response to ROS are also important in the pathogenesis of different liver diseases

[8]. Food contains diverse phytochemicals including antioxidant molecules that may play an important role in preserving the liver from oxidative stress-induced diseases. The consumption of antioxidant-rich foods may help enhance the antioxidant capacity of the body and would therefore reduce the risk of liver damage or may induce healing quickly [9]. A number of phytochemicals like naringenin, quercetin, curcumin, resveratrol, silymarin, carotenoids (*i.e.* lycopene, lutein, β-carotene, β-cryptoxanthin) present in edible plants also exhibit potent ROS scavenging effect. Further, pre-clinical/clinical studies indicated that these phytochemicals act via different mechanisms like reducing lipid accumulation, reducing insulin resistance, maintaining oxidative stress, and decreasing inflammatory cytokine generation and exhibit their beneficial effect in different liver disorders [8 - 10]. This chapter mainly focused on the beneficial effect of edible plants in liver disorders.

HEPATOPROTECTIVE VALUE OF EDIBLE PLANTS

Edible plants are also considered an important source of phytoconstituents with hepatoprotective activity. Plants are an important source of hepatoprotective activity and among them, edible plants could play an important role in protecting the liver from injury caused by oxidative stress, microorganisms, or other exogenous substances. A number of investigations reported the beneficial effects of edible plants or plant parts in liver diseases. Many vegetables, fruits, and spices have been investigated for their hepatoprotective activity in pre-clinical studies (Table **1**). A study on experimental animals showed that the plants/plant parts positively ameliorated liver enzymes like SGPT, SGPOT and other parameters. Further, these extracts enhanced the level of endogenous antioxidants and inhibited lipid peroxidation [11 - 19].

Table 1. Edible plants with hepatoprotective activity

Common Name	Plant name & Family	Edible Part	Model used	Parameter screened	Image
Pomelo / Grape Fruit	*Citrus paradisi* (Rutaceae)	Fruit	dimethylnitrosamine (DMN)-induced hepatic damage	ALAT, ASAT, ALP, and bilirubin, albumin, MDA	

(Table 1) cont.....

Common Name	Plant name & Family	Edible Part	Model used	Parameter screened	Image
Large Cranberry / American Cranberry / Bearberry	*Vaccinium macrocarpon* (Ericaceae)	Fruit	DMN-induced hepatic Lesions	Serum ALAT, ASAT, ALP, and Bilirubin, serum albumin and total protein levels, MDA	
Common Grape Vine	*Vitis vinifera* (Vitaceae)	Fruit	Ethanol- induced hepatic damage	ASAT, ALAT, GGT, LDH, MDA	
Fig Opuntia / Prickly Pear	*Opuntia ficus-indica* (Cactaceae)	Fruit	Chlorpyrifos induced hepatic damage	ALAT, ASAT, ALP, LDH, cholesterol, and albumin,	

(Table 1) cont.....

Common Name	Plant name & Family	Edible Part	Model used	Parameter screened	Image
Onion	*Allium cepa L* Amaryllidaceae	Bulb, Tender Leaves	CCl$_4$ Ethyl acetate, Paracetamol, Cadmium -induced hepatotoxicity	SGOT, SGPT, ALP and bilirubin, ALT, AST	
Garlic	*Allium sativum L* (Amaryllidaceae)	Bulbs	Paracetamol, Alloxan, Isoniazid, lead induced Hepatotoxicity	ALT, AST, and ALP	
Elephant Foot Yam	*Amorphophallus paeoniifolius* (Araceae)	Tubers	Paracetamol induced hepatic injury	SGOT, SGPT, SALP and Serum bilirubin	

(Table 1) cont.....

Common Name	Plant name & Family	Edible Part	Model used	Parameter screened	Image
Winter Melon, Ash Gourd	*Benincasa hispida* (Cucurbitaceae)	Fruits	Diclofenac-sodium induced hepatic injury	SGOT, SGPT, ALP	
Beet	*Beta vulgaris* (Amaranthaceae)	Root	CCl_4 induced hepatic damage	AST, ALT, ALP, total protein and bilirubin	
Mustard	*Brassica juncea* (Brassicaceae)	Seed	CCl_4 induced hepatic damage	AST, ALT, ALP, and GGT	

(Table 1) cont.....

Common Name	Plant name & Family	Edible Part	Model used	Parameter screened	Image
Cabbage	*Brassica oleracea* (Brassicaceae)		Simvastatin induced hepatotoxicity	SGPT, SGOT, ALP, Serum bilirubin and decrease in Total proteins	
Papaya	*Carica papaya* (Caricaceae)	Fruit	CCl_4, Paracetamol and Thioacetamide, induced hepatic damage	AST, ALT, ALP, total bilirubin and GGTP	
Lemon	*Citrus limon* (Rutaceae)	Fruits / Leaves	CCl_4 induced hepatic damage	total and direct bilirubin, MDA	
Colocasia	*Colocasia antiquorum* (Araceae)	Corms	Paracetamol and CCl_4 intoxicated rats	SGOT, SGPT	

(Table 1) cont.....

Common Name	Plant name & Family	Edible Part	Model used	Parameter screened	Image
Taro	*Colocasia esculenta* (Araceae)	Leaf Juice	Paracetamol and CCl_4 induced hepatic damage	AST, ALT, ALP	
Coriander	*Coriandrum sativum* (Apiaceae)	Seed	Lead nitrate induced oxidative stress and tissue damage in the liver	AST, ALT, ACP, ALP and total cholesterol	
Turmeric	*Curcuma longa* (Zingiberaceae)	Rhizome	CCl_4 induced hepatic damage	SGOT, SGPT and bilirubin level	

(Table 1) cont.....

Common Name	Plant name & Family	Edible Part	Model used	Parameter screened	Image
Cumin	*Cuminum cymimum* (Apiaceae)	Seed	Profenofos induced hepatic damage	SGPT, SGOT and serum bilirubin	
Carrot	*Daucus carota sativus* (Apiaceae)	Leaf And Root	CCl_4 induced hepatic damage	SGOT, SGPT, ALP, LDH,GLDH, Serum bilirubin, Hepatic 5'-nucleotidase, ACP, Acid ribonuclease, Succinic dehydrogenase, Glucose-6-phosphatase, Cytochrome P-450.	
Bottle Gourd	*Lagenaria siceraria* (Cucurbitaceae)	Fruits	CCl_4 induced hepatic damage	Total bilirubin, Serum protein, ALP, ALT, AST	

(Table 1) cont.....

Common Name	Plant name & Family	Edible Part	Model used	Parameter screened	Image
Ridge Gourd	*Luffa acutangula* (Cucurbitaceae)	Fruits	CCl4 & Rifampicin induced hepatic damage	AST, ALT, ALP and LDH total protein	
Horse Gram	*Macrotyloma uniflorum* (Fabaceae)	Seed	Paracetamol & D-Galactosamine induced hepatic damage	SGPT, SGOT, ALP, Bilirubin	
Mint	*Mentha arvensis* (Lamiaceae)	Leaves And Whole Plant	CCl₄ & Ethanol induced hepatic damage	SGPT, SGOT, ALP, Total Bilirubin, Total Protein, Tissue Glycogen	

(Table 1) cont.....

Common Name	Plant name & Family	Edible Part	Model used	Parameter screened	Image
Bitter Gourd	*Momordica charantia* (Cucurbitaceae)	Fruits	Acetaminophen induced hepatic damage	ALT, AST, ALP, LDH	
Drumstick	*Moringa oleifera* (Moringaceae)	Leaves, Pod	CCl_4 induced hepatic damage	SGPT, SGOT, Total Bilirubin, Direct Bilirubin	
Curry Leaf	*Murraya koenigii* Rutaceae	Leaves	Ethanol induced hepatic damage	GSH, LPO, CAT, SOD, Total protein	

(Table 1) cont.....

Common Name	Plant name & Family	Edible Part	Model used	Parameter screened	Image
Banana	*Musa paradisiaca* (Musaceae)	Fruits	Paracetamol induced hepatic damage	ALT, AST,Total protein, TG, cholesterol, GSH, LPO	
Sesame	*Sesamum indicum* (Pedaliaceae)	Seed	Paracetamol induced hepatic damage	SGOT, SGPT, ALP, ACP Total Biluribin	

(Table 1) cont.....

Common Name	Plant name & Family	Edible Part	Model used	Parameter screened	Image
Tomato	*Solanum lycopersicum* (Solanaceae)	Fruits	CCl$_4$ induced hepatic damage	AST, ALT, ALP, Total bilirubin	
Spinach	*Spinacia oleracea* (Amaranthaceae)	Leaves	CCl$_4$ induced hepatic damage	GGT, AST, ALT, ALP, serum- bilirubin,	
Black Gram	*Vigna mungo* (Fabaceae)	Seed	Ethanol induced hepatic damage	SGOT, SGPT, ALP, Total Biluribin	

(Table 1) cont.....

Common Name	Plant name & Family	Edible Part	Model used	Parameter screened	Image
Ginger	*Zingiber officinale* (Zingiberaceae)	Rhizome	Paracetamol induced hepatic damage	AST, ALT, ALP, Total bilirubin	
Broccoli	*Brassica oleracea L* (Brassicaceae)	Leaves	Simvastatin induced hepatic damage	SGOT and SGPT, ALP, Cholesterol, bilirubin, Serum total protein	
Spiny Gourd	*Momordica dioica* (Cucurbitaceae)	Fruit	CCl$_4$ induced hepatic damage	SGOT, SGPT, Total Bilirubin, ALP	

(Table 1) cont.....

Common Name	Plant name & Family	Edible Part	Model used	Parameter screened	Image
Celery	*Apium graveolens L.* (Apiaceae)	Whole Plant	Cholesterol rich diet	AST, ALT, ALP, TG, Cholesterol, HDL, VLDL, LDL	

Alanine Transaminase: ALAT; Aspartate Transaminase: ASAT; Alkaline Phosphatase: ALP; Aspartate Aminotransferase: AST; Alanine Aminotransferase: ALT; Malondialdehyde: MDA; Gamma-Glutamyl Transferase: GGT; Lactate Dehydrogenase: LDH; Serum Glutamic Oxaloacetic Transaminase: SGOT; Serum Glutamic Pyruvic Transaminase: SGPT; Serum Alkaline Phosphatase: SALP; Gamma-Glutamyl Transferase:GGT; Gamma-Glutamate Transpeptidase: GGTP; Average Total Acid Phosphatase: ACP; Glutamate Dehydrogenase: GLDH; Reduced Glutathione: GSH; Catalase: CAT, Superoxide Dismutase: SOD; Lipid Peroxide: LPO; Triglycerides: TG; High Density Lipoprotein: HDL; Very Low Density Lipoprotein: VLDL; Low Density Lipoprotein: LDL.

POSSIBLE HEPATOPROTECTIVE MECHANISM OF PHYTOCONS-TITUENT / PHYTOMEDICINE

Edible plants with hepatoprotective activity contain diverse phytochemicals that have antioxidant and hepatoprotective activity (Illustrated in Figure 1). Different phytoconstituents like curcumin, catechin, rutin, myristicin, fumaric acid, silybin, picroside, kutkoside, glycyrrihizin, silymarin, apigenin, *etc.* are frequently available in plants with hepatoprotective activity and also exhibited potent antioxidant activity [20]. In the 21st century, the paradigm shifted towards using food as a medicine and edible plants to manage or avert hepatic disorder. Silymerin was found to possess antioxidant, anti-inflammatory, and antifibrotic activity while exhibited membrane stabilizing angiogenesis regenerative property. Curcumin, is another phytoconstituent well-recognised for its anti-inflammatory, anticancer, and antioxidant activities. Resveratrol is an important phytoconstituent found in grapes and barriers exhibiting antiaging, regenerative, anti-inflammatory, and antioxidant activity. Apigenin can check lipid accumulation, amplify endogenous antioxidants and inhibit lipid peroxidation. Oxidative stress is an important mechanism that can cause the destruction of hepatic cells and can stimulate the production of inflammatory or proinflammatory mediators like activation of TGF-β stimulation involved in fibrosis. Increased generation of free radicals can cause increased ER stress, lipid peroxidation, mitochondrial dysfunction, apoptosis, DNA damage, NF-kB inflammation, *etc.* Different inflammatory and proinflammatory mediators like TNF, IL1β, IL6, COX, VCAM-1, TGFβ, IL8, *etc.* are involved in fibrosis, dysfunction of endothelial cells, *etc.* Inhibition of silent information regulators T1 (SIRT1), adenosine--monophosphate activated protein kinase (AMPK), depletion of endogenous antioxidants, and the activation of caspase-3 are also involved in the pathogenesis of liver disorder. Phytochemicals positively ameliorate such conditions and prevent damage to hepatic cells [21]. Phenolic compounds stabilize the cell membrane and avert oxidative stress, and they also inhibit excessive formation of inflammatory cytokines (*i.e.* TNF, TFGβ, IL2, IL6, IL8) and enhance the level of enzymatic (*i.e.* SOD, CAT, GPX, GR) and non-enzymatic (*i.e.* GSH) antioxidants. The liver is the central organ for the inactivation of xenobiotics and different Cytochrome P450 are expressed in the liver that can generate free radicals [22]. Luteolin has sbeen found to modulate the expression of drug-metabolizing enzymes, NADPH: NQO1 and aldo-keto reductase. Luteolin also inhibits hepatic lipogenesis and improves hepatosteatosis. Genistein inhibits NFkB and AMPK signalling, exhibits antifibrotic activity, and inhibits TGF-β1 expression. A number of phenolic compounds also act as regulators of gene expression which may be linked with their hepatoprotective effect. Apigenin has been found to down regulate Nrf2-signallig and up-regulate BCL-2 apoptotic pathway. Caffeic acid modulates the expression of hepatic carcinoma factor known as Keap1 and enhances the expression of HO-1(anti-oxidative signal). Curcumin suppresses Akt activation and ameliorates the expression of Nrf2, SOD, CAT, and GSH. Epicatechin down regulates liver enzymes (SGOT, SGPT). Ferulic acid inhibits gene expression that is related to extra cellular matrix and also causes the disruption of Smad signalling pathway. Genistein down regulates different genes including SREBP-1C, liver X receptor, retinoid X receptor, and PPAR-gama [22, 23].

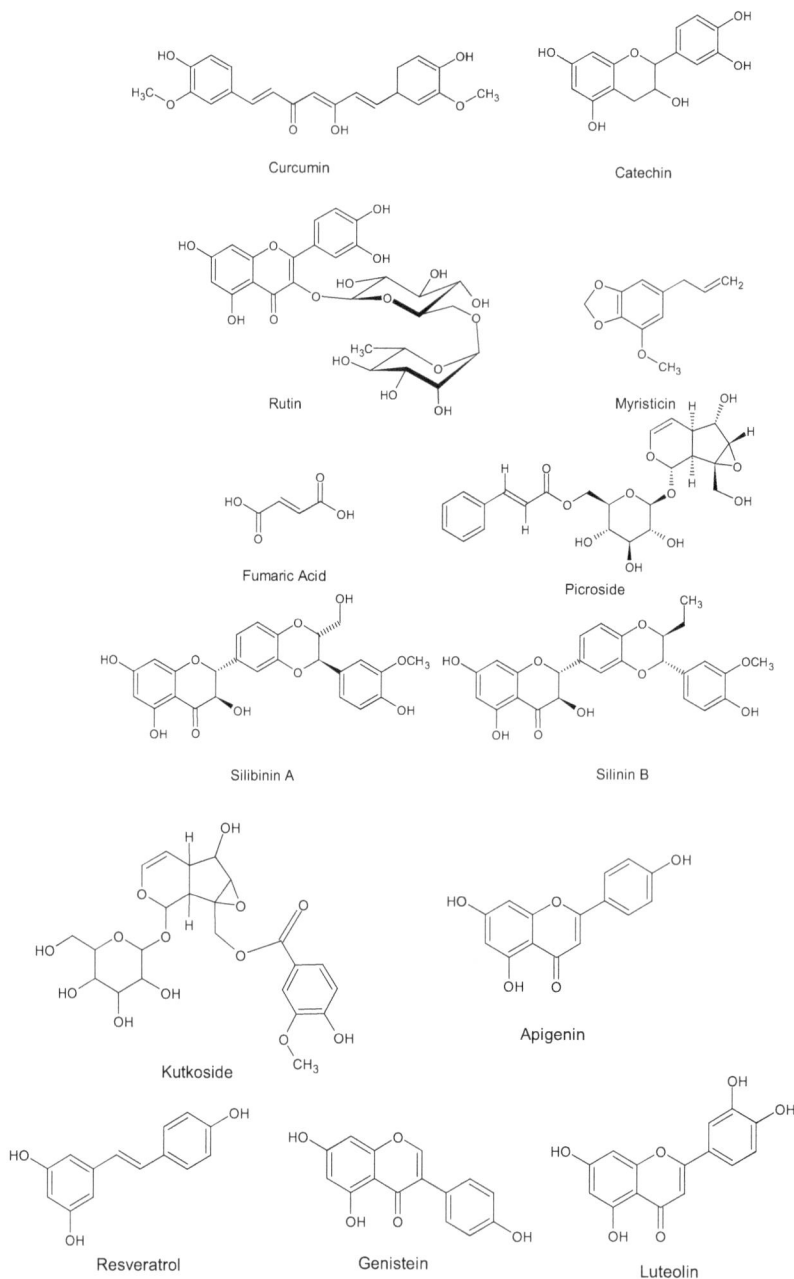

Fig. (1). Structure of phytochemicals from edible plants and spices with hepatoprotective potential

Many phytoconstituents has been studied extensively and these phytoconstituents may confer hepatoprotective activity through a number of mechanisms majorly linked with their antioxidant, anti-inflammatory, and cytoprotective activity (Fig. **2**).

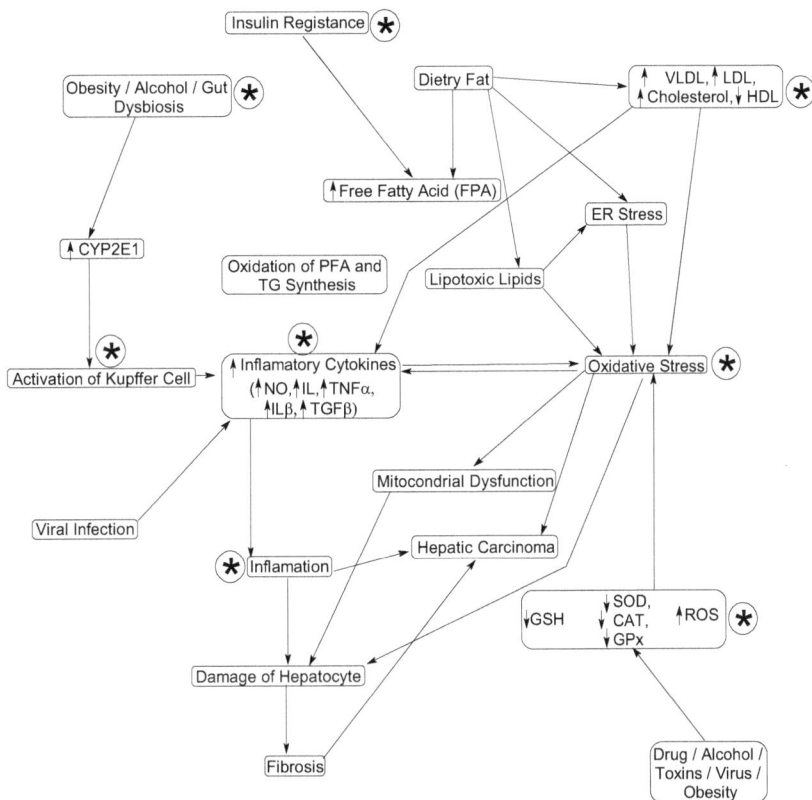

Fig. (2). Common pathogenesis involved in the different liver disorder and site of action of hepatoprotective phytochemicals (* indicates the site of action of phytochemicals)

CONCLUSION

In recent times, there is a rise in the number of mortality and morbidity associated with different liver disorders. Plants rich in bioactive phytochemicals with antioxidant, antiviral, and anti-inflammatory activities are considered alternatives in preventing and managing liver diseases. Effective management of liver disease by the dietary or herbal method is one of the important concepts of complementary and alternative medicine. Diverse phytochemicals have been found beneficial in liver disorders that act through different mechanisms. Edible whole plants, fruits, spices, and vegetables could offer better alternatives to the restricted therapeutic options that exist in the management or prevention of hepatic diseases. In general, this chapter enlisted few edible plants with hepatoprotective activity and highlighted the hepatoprotective mechanisms of phytochemicals present in such plants. Of course, a detailed study for evaluation of such leads, particularly through advanced pre-clinical and clinical studies, is necessary for the future.

REFERENCES

[1]   Moradi, M.T.; Asadi-Samani, M.; Bahmani, M.; Shahrani, M. Medicinal plants used for liver disorders based on the ethnobotanical documents of Iran: A review. *Int. J. Pharm. Tech. Res.,* **2016**, *9*, 407-415.

[2]   Lim, H.K.; Jeffrey, G.P.; Ramm, G.A.; Soekmadji, C. Pathogenesis of viral hepatitis-induced chronic liver disease: Role of extracellular vesicles. *Front. Cell. Infect. Microbiol.,* **2020**, *10*, 587628.
[http://dx.doi.org/10.3389/fcimb.2020.587628] [PMID: 33240824]

[3]   Marcellin, P.; Kutala, B.K. Liver diseases: A major, neglected global public health problem requiring urgent actions and large-scale screening. *Liver Int.,* **2018**, *38* 1, 2-6.
[http://dx.doi.org/10.1111/liv.13682] [PMID: 29427496]

[4]   Asrani, S.K.; Devarbhavi, H.; Eaton, J.; Kamath, P.S. Burden of liver diseases in the world. *J. Hepatol.,* **2019**, *70*(1), 151-171.
[http://dx.doi.org/10.1016/j.jhep.2018.09.014] [PMID: 30266282]

[5]   Balogh, J.; Victor, D., III; Asham, E.H.; Burroughs, S.G.; Boktour, M.; Saharia, A.; Li, X.; Ghobrial, M.; Monsour, H., Jr Hepatocellular carcinoma: A review. *J. Hepatocell. Carcinoma,* **2016**, *3*, 41-53.
[http://dx.doi.org/10.2147/JHC.S61146] [PMID: 27785449]

[6]   Osna, N.A.; Donohue, T.M., Jr; Kharbanda, K.K. Alcoholic liver disease: Pathogenesis and current management. *Alcohol Res.,* **2017**, *38*(2), 147-161.
[PMID: 28988570]

[7]   Sen, S.; Chakraborty, R. Food in Health Preservation and Promotion: A special focus on the interplay between oxidative stress and pro-oxidant/antioxidant. In: *Exploring the Nutrition and Health Benefits of Functional Foods,* 1st ed; Shekhar, H.U.; Howlader, Z.H.; Kabir, Y., Eds.; IGI Global: USA, **2016**; pp. 265-300.

[8]   Li, S.; Tan, H.Y.; Wang, N.; Zhang, Z.J.; Lao, L.; Wong, C.W.; Feng, Y. The role of oxidative stress and antioxidants in liver diseases. *Int. J. Mol. Sci.,* **2015**, *16*(11), 26087-26124.
[http://dx.doi.org/10.3390/ijms161125942] [PMID: 26540040]

[9]   Appak-Baskoy, S.; Cengiz, M.; Teksoy, O.; Ayhanci, A. Dietary antioxidants in experimental models of liver diseases. In: *Strawberry-Pre-and Post-Harvest Management Techniques for Higher Fruit Quality*; IntechOpen, **2019**.
[http://dx.doi.org/10.5772/intechopen.83485]

[10]   Elvira-Torales, L.I.; García-Alonso, J.; Periago-Castón, M.J. Nutritional importance of carotenoids and their effect on liver health: A review. *Antioxidants,* **2019**, *8*(7), 229-252.
[http://dx.doi.org/10.3390/antiox8070229] [PMID: 31330977]

[11]   Madrigal-Santillán, E.; Madrigal-Bujaidar, E.; Álvarez-González, I.; Sumaya-Martínez, M.T.; Gutiérrez-Salinas, J.; Bautista, M.; Morales-González, Á.; García-Luna y González-Rubio, M.; Aguilar-Faisal, J.L.; Morales-González, J.A. Review of natural products with hepatoprotective effects. *World J. Gastroenterol.,* **2014**, *20*(40), 14787-14804.
[http://dx.doi.org/10.3748/wjg.v20.i40.14787] [PMID: 25356040]

[12]   Ahmed, M.F.; Rao, A.S.; Ahemad, S.R.; Ibrahim, M. Protective effect of *Brassica oleracea L. var. capitata* against simvastatin induced hepatotoxicity in rats. *Int Res J of Pharmaceuticals.,* **2012**, *2*, 91-97.

[13]   Maximas, H.; Rose, H.R.; Sudha, P.N.; Vinayagam, A.; Sudhakar, K. A review on hepatoprotective

activity of commonly consumed vegetables. *Pharm. Lett.,* **2013**, *5*, 290-304.

[14]   Kushwaha, S.K.; Jain, A.; Jain, A.; Gupta, V.B.; Patel, J.R. Hepatoprotective activity of the fruits of *Momordica dioica. Niger. J. Nat. Prod. Med.,* **2005**, *9*, 29-31.

[15]   Jaiswal, S.K.; Gupta, V.K.; Siddiqi, N.J.; Pandey, R.S.; Sharma, B. Hepatoprotective effect of *Citrus limon* fruit extract against carbofuran induced toxicity in wistar rats. *Zhongguo Shengwuzhipinxue Zazhi,* **2015**, *2015*, 1-10.

[16]   Subramanian, V. Hepatoprotective activity of *Brassica oleracea Italica* against carbon tetrachloride induced in albino rats. *J. Pharm. Res.,* **2011**, *4*, 1143-1144.

[17]   Belal, N.M. Hepatoprotective effect of feeding celery leaves mixed with chicory leaves and barley grains to hypercholestemic rats. *Asia Pac. J. Clin. Nutr.,* **2011**, *3*, 12-24.

[18]   Islam, M.; Islam, M.S.; Zannah, S.; Rashid, M. Combination Therapy of *Momordica charantia* Linn. (Bitter Melon) with antihyperglycemic agent gives increased antioxidative and hepatoprotective actions in alloxan-induced diabetic rats. *Bangladesh Pharmaceutical Journal,* **2019**, *22*(1), 34-40. [http://dx.doi.org/10.3329/bpj.v22i1.40023]

[19]   Aćimović, M.G.; Milić, N.B.; Milic, N.B. Perspectives of the *Apiaceae* hepatoprotective effects : A review. *Nat. Prod. Commun.,* **2017**, *12*(2), 1934578X1701200. [http://dx.doi.org/10.1177/1934578X1701200241] [PMID: 30428236]

[20]   Jadon, A. Medicinal plants as hepatoprotective agents in Indian systems of medicine: A review. *Integrated Research Advances.,* **2018**, *5*(2), 36-41.

[21]   Farghali, H.; Canová, N.K.; Zakhari, S. Hepatoprotective properties of extensively studied medicinal plant active constituents: Possible common mechanisms. *Pharm. Biol.,* **2015**, *53*(6), 781-791. [http://dx.doi.org/10.3109/13880209.2014.950387] [PMID: 25489628]

[22]   Saha, P.; Talukdar, A.D.; Nath, R.; Sarker, S.D.; Nahar, L.; Sahu, J.; Choudhury, M.D. Role of natural phenolics in hepatoprotection: A mechanistic review and analysis of regulatory network of associated genes. *Front. Pharmacol.,* **2019**, *10*, 509-534. [http://dx.doi.org/10.3389/fphar.2019.00509] [PMID: 31178720]

[23]   Domitrović, R.; Potočnjak, I. A comprehensive overview of hepatoprotective natural compounds: Mechanism of action and clinical perspectives. *Arch. Toxicol.,* **2016**, *90*(1), 39-79. [http://dx.doi.org/10.1007/s00204-015-1580-z] [PMID: 26377694]

CHAPTER 7

Hepatoprotective Phytochemicals: Isolation and Characterization from Plant Extracts

Biresh Kumar Sarkar[1,*], **Dhrubajyoti Sarkar**[2], **Faruk Alam**[3] and **Durgaprasad Kemisetti**[3]

[1] *Central Ayurveda Research Institute, CCRAS, Ministry of AYUSH, 4-CN Block, Sector- V, Bidhannagar, Kolkata-700091, India*

[2] *Faculty of Pharmaceutical Science, Assam Down Town University, Sankar Medhab Path Panikhaiti Guwahati 781026, India*

[3] *Faculty of Pharmaceutical Science, Assam Down Town University, Panikhaiti, Guwahati, Assam-781026, India*

Abstract: The liver is the body's primary organ responsible for metabolism and excretion. Oxidation, reduction, hydration, condensation, hydrolysis, conjugation, and isomerization are some of the metabolic routes used by the human liver to metabolise chemicals. Any of the aforementioned processes can be disrupted, resulting in liver cell damage or hepatotoxicity, which can lead to a variety of disorders. These disorders are linked to increased death rates over the world. Medicines, chemicals, dietary changes, and herb-induced liver injury via hepatotoxins can all cause hepatotoxicity. A number of herbal and herbomineral preparations are available in Ayurveda, the traditional Indian Medicine, which has been investigated for their hepatoprotective potential to treat different types of liver disorders. The present review is focused on different herbal plants that have the potential to cure hepatotoxicity.

Keywords: Herbal plants, Hepatotoxicity, Liver diseases, Herbal drugs, Indian Herb, Phytochemical.

INTRODUCTION

The liver is one of the body's most important organs. Its activity is linked to several critical activities, such as metabolism, secretion, and storage space, and it plays an important role in controlling various physiological processes. Many researchers have studied its ability to detoxify endogenous (waste metabolites) and/or exogenous (toxic chemicals) substances of organisms, as well as manufacture beneficial agents, since the 1970s [1 - 4].

* **Corresponding author Biresh Kumar Sarkar:** Central Ayurveda Research Institute, CCRAS, Ministry of AYUSH, 4-CN Block, Sector- V, Bidhannagar, Kolkata- 700091, India; E-mail: bireshsarkar@gmail.com

Sachin Kumar Jain, Ram Kumar Sahu, Priyanka Soni, Vishal Soni & Shiv Shankar Shukla (Eds.)

The liver has a role in all biochemical activities, such as in growth, reproduction, delivering nutrition, and supplying energy to the body's organs. It also helps in the metabolism of carbohydrates and lipids, the production of bile, and the storage of vitamins [5]. Hepatic illnesses continue to be one of the most serious dangers to public health, and they are a concern all over the world [4, 6]. Hepatic disease is a term that refers to an injury to the cells, tissues, structure, or function of the liver. It can be caused by biological factors (bacteria, viruses, and parasites), autoimmune diseases (immune hepatitis, primary biliary cirrhosis), or the action of different chemicals (some drugs), toxic chemicals [carbon tetrachloride (CCl4), thioacetamide, dimethylnitrosamine (DMN), D-galactosamine/lipopolysaccharide (GalN/LPS)], and, without a doubt, excessive alcohol intake [7 - 9]. Despite tremendous developments in contemporary medicine, no fully effective medications exist that stimulate hepatic activity, provide total organ protection, or help in the regeneration of hepatic cells [10, 11]. Furthermore, certain medicines might cause side effects. As a result, alternative medications for the treatment of hepatic illnesses must be identified, with the goal of making these drugs more effective and less harmful. The usage of some plants and the consumption of various fruits have played important roles in human health care. Around 80% of the world's population relies on traditional medicine for treatment [4, 9], which is mostly based on plant components. Various scientific investigations of medicinal plants and the consumption of fruits have revealed that the properties responsible for their beneficial effects can be attributed to the presence of biologically active chemical compounds or substances called phytochemicals, which are supplementary nutrients for life. In conclusion, research that has looked at the impact that various phytochemicals have on health may be found. The following are some of the most often mentioned examples: (1) The vinca alkaloids (vincristine, vinblastine, and vindesine); (2) The betalain pigments (betanin and indicaxanthine); (3) Anthocyanins (cranberries); and (4) Resveratrol; all of these have been studied for their cancer-fighting potential [4, 12 - 14]. All therapeutic plants, as well as the consumption of certain fruits, have different impacts on biological systems. Although a few studies have looked at their hepatoprotective properties, the vast bulk of research has focused on their sedative, analgesic, antipyretic, cardioprotective, antibacterial, antiviral, antiprotozoal, and anticarcinogenic properties [15]. In addition to these studies, there is a long history of experiential confirmation on the use of natural remedies for the treatment of hepatic diseases, and this field has emerged as an innovative field of research, with the primary goal of analysing the consumption of traditional fruits and medicinal plants by a large number of people, as well as the various phytochemicals extracted from these foods. Chemical substances found in liver-protective fruits and plants include phenols, coumarins, lignans, essential oils, monoterpenes, glycosides, alkaloids, carotenoids, flavonoids, organic acids, and xanthenes [16]. The goal was to compile data from studies on some fruits and plants that are commonly consumed by humans and have been shown to have hepatoprotective properties, as well as an analysis of a resin and some phytochemicals extracted from fruits, plants, yeasts, and algae that have been tested in various hepatotoxicity models [17 - 20]. When it comes to detoxifying the many poisons found in food, beverages, drugs, and the environment, the liver can take the most abuse. Pre-existing liver illness, age, female sex, and heredity are only a few of the risk factors that might lead to hepatic drug harm. The liver, as the primary site of metabolism, plays a critical role in the detoxification of many toxins consumed and/or created during food absorption [1 - 3]. To prevent toxins from accessing other bodily systems, the liver filters all blood from the digestive tract before passing it on to the rest of the body [4]. It controls practically all of the body's processes by utilising several metabolic pathways for energy generation, metabolism, and reproduction [5]. The liver also produces a variety of complement systems and proteins that aid the immune system [6]. As a result, a functioning liver is essential for a healthy person.

Causes of Liver Diseases

Due to food choices, alcohol use, poor cleanliness, uncontrolled drug use, and smoking, liver problems are the most common health concern in underdeveloped nations. Non-inflammatory, inflammatory, and degenerative liver illnesses are all possible. Because of hepatic insufficiency, high levels of plasma total cholesterol (LDL-C) and triacylglycerols (TGs) are linked to an increased risk of atherosclerosis and cardiovascular disease [7, 8]. Hepatotoxicity is caused by a variety of toxins such as carbon tetrachloride (CCl4), thioacetamide, acute or chronic alcohol intake, various illnesses such as hepatitis A, B, and C, and medications, the latter of which is the most commonly reported. Free radical generations with alcohol use result in the development of hepatitis, leading to cirrhosis [21].

Role of Medicinal Plants in Hepatotoxicity

Plant materials have been employed in Ayurveda to protecting the liver from various poisons and dietary factors. As a result, herbal treatments have grown in popularity in recent years due to their safety and potential to cure ailments. These drugs are also incredibly cost-effective when used for a long time. Many medicinal plants found in various areas of India have been identified as hepatoprotective medications and are widely utilised to treat liver diseases. Hepatoprotective action may be found in a variety of plants and polyherbal preparations. Hepatoprotective action has been claimed for around 160 phytoconstituents and other phytochemicals [10]. Over 87 plants are utilised in

India, with 33 of them being trademarked and having exclusive multi-ingredient plant compositions [22]. To emphasise the importance of their use, we looked at a variety of well-known herbal plants with hepatoprotective properties.

Isolation and Characterization from Plant Extracts

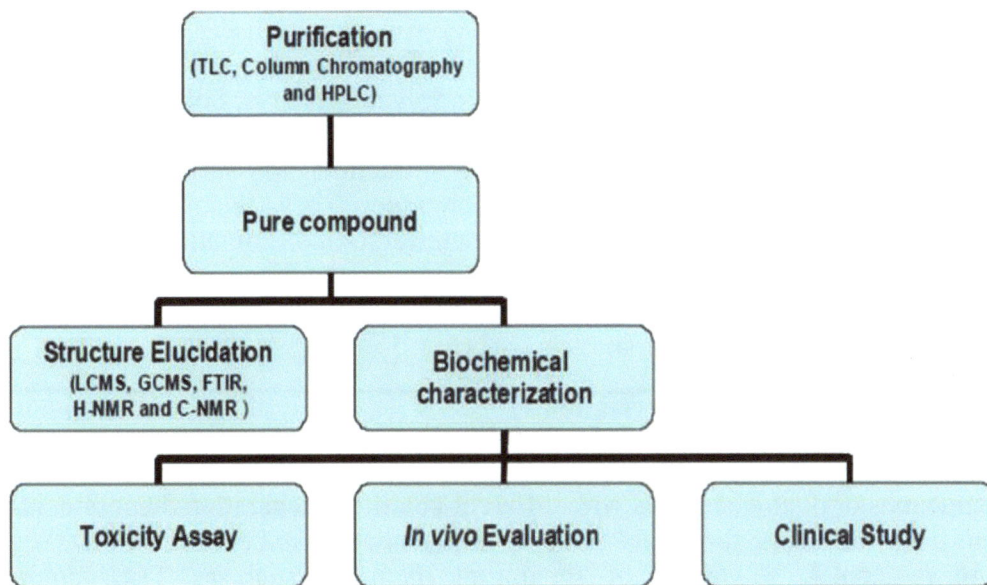

Fig. 1. A brief summary of the general approaches in extraction, isolation, and characterization of bioactive compounds from plants extract.

Extraction

Because it is important to separate the desired chemical components from plant materials for further severance and characterization, extraction is a critical initial step in the investigation of medicinal plants. Pre-washing, drying of plant materials or freeze drying, grinding to get a homogeneous sample, frequently enhancing the kinetics of analytic extraction, and boosting the contact of the sample façade with the solvent system were all part of the fundamental process. Suitable measures must be taken to ensure that possible active ingredients are not lost, altered, or destroyed during the extraction of plant materials. If the plant was chosen based on its traditional applications [22], then the extract must be prepared according to the traditional healer's instructions in order to duplicate the traditional 'herbal' medication as nearly as possible. The choice of solvent solution is mostly determined by the type of bioactive molecule being studied. To extract the bioactive ingredient from natural sources, many solvent systems are available. Polar solvents such as methanol, ethanol, or ethyl-acetate are used to extract hydrophilic substances. Dichloromethane, or a 1:1 combination of dichloromethane and methanol, is used to extract more lipophilic substances. Hexane extraction has been utilised to remove chlorophyll in some cases [23]. Because the target molecules might range from being non-polar to polar and thermally labile, the suitability of extraction procedures must be evaluated. For the extraction of plant materials, several procedures such as sonification, heating under reflux, soxhlet extraction, and others are often utilised [24 - 26]. Plant extracts can also be made by macerating or percolating fresh green plants or powdered plant material in water or organic solvent systems. Solid-phase micro-extraction, supercritical-fluid extraction, pressurized-liquid extraction, microwave-assisted extraction, solid-phase extraction, and surfactant-mediated procedures are other modern extraction techniques. These include reductions in organic solvent consumption and sample deterioration, elimination of additional sample clean-up, and improvement in extraction competence, selectivity, and/or kinetics. The ease with which these processes may be automated also promotes their use for extracting plant materials [27] (Fig. **1**).

Identification and Characterization

Because plant extracts usually contain a mixture of several types of bioactive compounds or phytochemicals with different polarities, separating them remains a significant challenge for bioactive compound detection and classification. To get pure molecules, a variety of separation methods, such as TLC, column chromatography, flash chromatography, Sephadex chromatography, and HPLC, are commonly utilised in the extraction of these bioactive chemicals. The structure and biological activity of the pure chemicals are then determined. Besides that, non-chromatographic techniques such as immunoassay, which use monoclonal antibodies (MAbs), phytochemical screening assay, and Fourier-transform infrared spectroscopy (FTIR), can also be used to get and make possible the identification of bioactive compounds [28].

CHROMATOGRAPHIC TECHNIQUES

Thin-layer chromatography (TLC) and Bio-autographic methods

TLC is a straightforward, fast, and cost-effective method for determining how many components are present in a mixture. When the Rf of a compound is compared to the Rf of a known compound, TLC is also used to retain the identification of a chemical in a mixture. Additional tests include spraying phytochemical screening reagents, which change the colour depending on the phytochemicals included in a plant extract, or observing the plate under UV light. This method has also been used to verify the purity and originality of isolated chemicals. Bio-autography is a method for determining bioactive compounds with antibacterial activity from plant extracts. TLC bioautographic approaches combine chromatographic separation with in situ activity measurement, making it easier to locate and isolate active elements in a combination. Detecting anti-microbial components in extracts chromatographed on a TLC layer has traditionally been done using the growth embarrassment of bacteria. This technology has been deemed the most effective method for detecting antimicrobial chemicals [29].

Bio-autography uses three methods to locate antimicrobial activity on a chromatogram:

- Direct bio-autography, involves the microbe growing straight on a thin-layer chromatographic (TLC) plate.
- Contact bio-autography, where antimicrobial chemicals are transferred directly from the TLC plate to an inoculated agar plate, and agar overlay bio-autography, in which a seeded agar medium is put directly into the TLC plate [30, 31].
- Inhibition zones created on TLC plates using one of the foregoing bio-autographic techniques will be used to see the position of the bioactive molecule with antimicrobial activity in the TLC fingerprint using R_f values [32].

The same stationary and mobile phases were used to construct preparative TLC plates with a thickness of 1mm, with the goal of isolating the bioactive components that demonstrate antimicrobial action in addition to the test strain. The substance was eluted from the silica with ethanol or methanol after these spots were scraped off the plates. Using the preparative chromatography procedure described above, eluted samples were further purified. Finally, HPLC, LCMS, and GCMS were used to identify the components. Its usefulness is restricted to microorganisms that easily grow on TLC plates, despite its great sensitivity. Other issues include the requirement to completely remove residual low-volatile solvents, including n-BuOH, trifluoroacetic acid, and ammonia, as well as the diffusion of active chemicals from the stationary phase into the agar layer [33 - 35]. Because bio-autography allows researchers to pinpoint an extract's antimicrobial activity on a chromatogram, it facilitates the quick discovery of novel antimicrobial agents using bioassay-guided isolation. When compared to the traditional disc diffusion approach, the bioautography agar method has several advantages. It utilises a much less amount of material. Hence, it can be used for bioassay-guided isolation of compounds. Secondly, since the crude extract is determined into its dissimilar components, this method simplifies the process of identification and isolation of the bioactive compounds [36].

High-Performance Liquid Chromatography

For the separation of natural compounds, high-performance liquid chromatography (HPLC) is a flexible, robust, and frequently used technology [37]. This methodology is now gaining favour among many analytical techniques as the preferred method for fingerprinting studies for herbal plant quality control [38]. In order to adequately describe the active ingredient, natural products are usually separated after a biological experiment evaluates a relatively crude extract. The biologically active item is frequently only a small component in the extract, and HPLC's resolving capacity is excellent for quickly processing such multicomponent samples on both an analytical and practical level. A solvent supply pump, a sample introduction tool such as an auto-sampler or manual injection valve, an analytical column, a guard column, a detector, and a recorder or printer are now included in many benchtop HPLC equipment. Chemical separations may be performed using HPLC by making use of the fact that different compounds migrate at different rates depending on the column and mobile phase. The choice of the stationary phase and movable phase determines the quantity or degree of separation. In general, an isocratic system (a single, unchanging mobile phase system) may be used to identify and separate phytochemicals [39]. If more than one sample component is being examined and their retention differs significantly under the circumstances used, the gradient elution, in which the quantity of organic solvent to water is changed over time, may be appealing. The process of separating or extracting the target chemical from other (potentially structurally similar) molecules or impurities using HPLC is known as the purification of the compound of interest. Under particular chromatographic conditions, each component should have a feature peak. The chromatographer may set the conditions, such as the right mobile phase, flow rate, detectors, and columns, to achieve the best separation depending on what has to be separated and how closely related the samples are. Compound identification by HPLC is an important aspect of every HPLC test. A detector must be chosen before any chemical may be recognised by HPLC. A separation assay must be established after the detector has been chosen and configured to optimal detection parameters. The assay parameters should be set so that a clear peak of the known sample may be seen on the chromatograph. The identifying peak should have a rational retention time and should be well separated from extraneous peaks at the detection levels at which the assay will be performed.

- UV detectors are the most common of all detectors because of their great sensitivity [40] and the fact that the majority of naturally occurring substances exhibit some UV absorption at short wavelengths (190-210 nm) [41].
- If a component of interest is only present in trace levels in the sample, UV

detection's great sensitivity is a plus. Other detection technologies, such as the diode array detector (DAD) linked with a mass spectrometer (MS), are being used to detect phytochemicals in addition to UV [42].

- For examining complicated plant extracts, liquid chromatography with mass spectrometry (LC/MS) is also a powerful approach [43 - 45]. When cyclic mass spectrometry (MSn) is used, it gives a wealth of information for the structural elucidation of the molecules. As a result, when a pure standard is unavailable, the combination of HPLC with MS allows for quick and exact identification of chemical components in medicinal plants [46].
- The way a crude source material is processed to generate a sample appropriate for HPLC analysis, as well as the solvent used to reconstitute the sample, can have a big impact on the overall outcome of natural product isolation.

The source material, such as dried powdered plant, must first be processed in order for the component of interest to be professionally fed into the solution. An organic solvent (e.g., methanol, chloroform) may be employed as the first extractant in the case of dried plant material, and solid material is subsequently removed by decanting off the extract by filtration after a time of maceration. After that, the filtrate is concentrated before being put into HPLC for separation. In the examination of crude extract, the use of guard columns is critical. Many natural product materials contain a noteworthy level of strongly binding components, such as chlorophyll and other endogenous materials that may, in the long term, cooperate with the presentation of analytical columns. Therefore, the guard columns will considerably protect the lifespan of the analytical columns.

NON-CHROMATOGRAPHIC TECHNIQUES

Immunoassay

Immunoassays, which utilise monoclonal antibodies to detect pharmaceuticals and low molecular weight natural bioactive chemicals, are becoming increasingly relevant in bioactive compound research. For receptor binding investigations, enzyme assays, and qualitative and quantitative analytical procedures have great specificity and sensitivity. In many circumstances, MAb-based enzyme-linked immunosorbent assays (ELISA) are more sensitive than traditional HPLC procedures. Hybridoma technology [47] is a technique for producing monoclonal antibodies in specialised cells.

The following steps are involved in the synthesis of monoclonal antibodies and plant medicines using hybridoma technology:

- A rabbit is immunised by administering certain plant medicines repeatedly in order to induce the formation of specific antibodies, which is aided by the growth of the appropriate B cells.

- A mouse or a rabbit can develop tumours.
- Spleen cells (which are rich in B cells and T cells) are cultivated separately from the other two types of animals. The spleen cells are cultivated separately and develop specific antibodies against the plant medicine, as well as myeloma cells, which create tumours.
- Polyethylene glycol is used to generate hybridoma formation by combining spleen cells with myeloma cells (PEG). In selective hypoxanthine aminopterin thymidine (HAT) media, the hybrid cells are fully developed.
- A preferred hybridoma is chosen for cloning and antibody manufacturing, as well as the development of plant medicine. Preparing single-cell colonies that will proliferate and can be utilised to test for antibody-producing hybridomas aids this progress.
- Selected hybridoma cells are cultivated in large quantities for the synthesis of monoclonal antibodies, as well as particular plant medicines.
- Monoclonal antibodies are utilised in enzyme-linked immunosorbent assays (ELISA) to evaluate similar medicines in plant extract combinations [48 - 52].

Phytochemical Screening Assay

Plant-derived chemicals are known as phytochemicals, and the phrase is typically used to describe the huge variety of secondary metabolic components and products present in plants. Phytochemical inquiry assay is a simple, rapid, and cost-effective procedure that allows researchers to respond quickly to various types of phytochemicals in combination and is a useful tool in bioactive compound analysis. Phytochemical screening can be done using the appropriate assays after obtaining the crude extract or active fraction from plant material.

Fourier-Transform Infrared Spectroscopy (FTIR)

The use of FTIR to categorise and recognise chemicals or functional groups (chemical bonds) present in an unidentified mixture of plant extracts has been proven [53, 54]. Furthermore, the FTIR spectra of pure substances are often so distinct that they resemble a chemical "fingerprint." The spectrum of an unknown molecule can be determined by comparing it to a library of known compounds for most common plant components. FTIR samples can be made in a variety of methods. Placing one drop of the sample between two plates of sodium chloride is the simplest method for liquid samples. Between the plates, the drop produces a thin film. Solid materials can be milled with potassium bromide (KBr) to form a thin pellet that can be examined. Solid samples can also be dissolved in a solvent like methylene chloride and then transferred to a single salt plate. After the solvent has evaporated, a thin coating of the unique substance is left on the plate.

Hepatoprotective Fruits

Grapefruit (Citrus paradisi)

Citrus paradisi is the scientific name for the grapefruit, which belongs to the genus Citrus in the Rutaceae family. The grapefruit was first planted on Barbados Island, but it is now grown in Mexico, Spain, Morocco, Israel, Jordan, South Africa, Brazil, Jamaica, and Asia [55]. In addition to being ingested as a common fruit or in juice to accompany other meals, it has been utilised as an antibacterial, antifungal, anti-inflammatory, antioxidant, and antiviral, as well as an astringent solution and an additional agent in several nations [56]. Grapefruit has been linked to cellular regeneration, cholesterol reduction, the detoxification process, heart health maintenance, rheumatoid arthritis, body weight control, and cancer prevention in studies undertaken over the last few decades [57 - 59]. Grapefruit juice is high in phytochemicals and nutrients, all contributing to a healthy diet. Vitamin C, folic acid, phenolic acid, potassium, calcium, iron, limonoids, terpenes, monoterpenes, and D-glucaric acid are all present in significant amounts. Beta-carotene and lycopene, antioxidants that the body can convert to vitamin A, are also found in the red and pink varieties [60] (Fig. **2**).

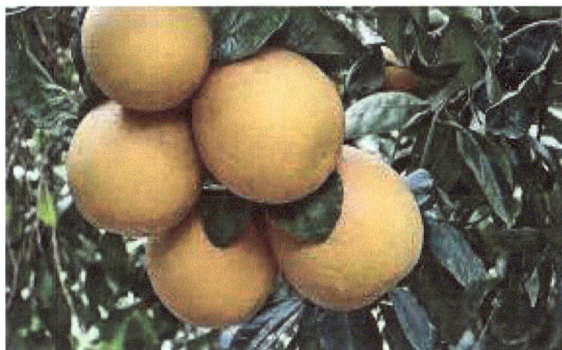

Fig. 2. *Grapefruit.*

On the other hand, the flavonoid with the greatest concentration is naringin, which humans metabolize into naringenin [61 - 65].

Blueberries/cranberries (Vaccinium spp.)

Berries account for a majority of the tiny, soft-fleshed, colorful fruits used in our diets. These fruits are consumed not just in their fresh and/or frozen form but also as processed foods such as canned fruits, yogurts, drinks, jams, and jellies. As a result, berry extracts have become more popular as a component in functional meals and nutritional supplements in recent years, which may or may not be combined with other colourful fruits, plants, and herbal extracts. The berry fruits that are usually consumed in North America include blackberries (*Rubus* spp.), black raspberries (*Rubus occidentalis*), red raspberries (*Rubus idaeus*), strawberries (*Fragaria X ananassa*), blueberries (*Vaccinium corymbosum*), and cranberries (*Vaccinium macrocarpon*) [66] (Fig. **3**).

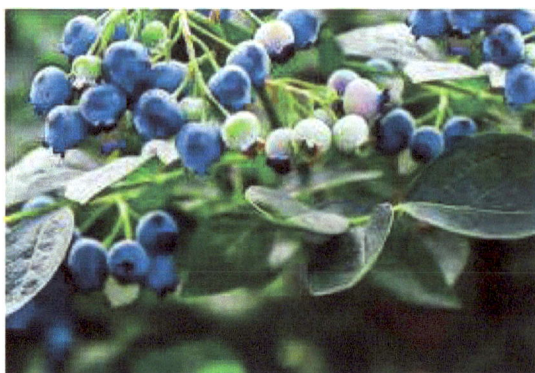

Fig. 3. *Vaccinium macrocarpon.*

Diverse research from Asia, Europe, New Zealand, Mexico, and North and South America was presented at the 2007 International Berry Health Advantages Symposium, establishing the probable benefits that may be acquired by eating an abundance of these fruits. In general, these advantages were reported in cardiovascular illnesses, neurological disorders, and other aging-related diseases, as well as obesity and several human malignancies (mainly esophageal and gastrointestinal). Diverse phenolic-type phytochemicals were established as the agents responsible for these biological features, with the following being emphasized.

Tannins [condensed tannins (proanthocyanidins) and hydrolyzable tannins (ellagitannins and gallotannins)]; Stilbenoids; and Phenolic acids [67]. The anthocyanins (pigments responsible for the berries' beautiful hues) have shown antioxidant, anticarcinogenic, and anti-inflammatory biological action [65 - 68], and are the most investigated of any of these chemicals.

Grape (Vitis vinifera L)

The grape (*Vitis vinifera*) is a woody climbing plant that may grow up to 30 metres in height when left to its own devices; however, owing to regular trimming, it is frequently reduced to a modest 1 metre shrub. The grape is a vine fruit that is edible and used as a raw material to make wine and other alcoholic drinks (Fig. **4**). Viticulture originated in Asia and Southeastern Europe, and as a result of this development, the grape has become an important part of human nutrition, and its cultivation has spread to the American and African continents. There are approximately 3000 varieties of grapes in the world, even though not all of these are uniformly esteemed. According to their final use, grapes are classified into two large groups:

1. Those designated for consumption with meals (table grapes);
2. Wine grapes, which are employed for the creation of wine [69].

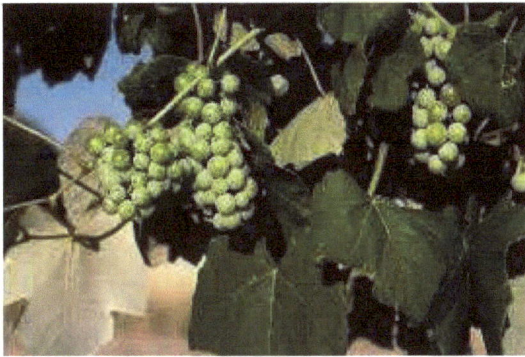

Fig. 4. *Vitis vinifera.*

The leaves, as well as the fruit, are an incredible source of vitamins, minerals, and other active elements; these components have been attributed to medical characteristics, which is why the grape has been classified as a drug food by several writers [37, 38]. Laxative, astringent, diuretic, cicatrisant, immunological stimulant, anti-inflammatory, and hypocholesterolemic properties, as well as chemopreventive activity against cardiovascular disease and several malignancies (primarily prostate and colon), have been derived from various components of this plant [39, 40].

Hepatoprotective Plants

Nopal (Cactus pear) and Tuna (Cactus pear fruit) "Opuntia ficus-indica."

The Cactaceae family, which includes plants from the genus *Opuntia*, is widely grown across the American continent, as well as in the Mediterranean, Europe, Asia, Africa, and Australia (Fig. **5**). The majority of *Opuntia spp.* have flat stems called pencas or cladodes (paddles), and the cactus pear (nopal) is the most common type [70]. The cactus pear fruits (tunas) or prickly pear fruits of this plant are oval berries with a large number of seeds and a semi-hard bark containing thorns, and they are divided into four groups based on their colours (red, purple, orange/yellow, and white). Usually, fruit with white pulp and green skin is ideal for utilization as food, and its conjugal production corresponds to nearly 95% of the total construction worldwide. Mexico is the primary producer of cactus pear fruits, representing more than 45% of global production; nevertheless, only 1.5% of this production is exported [71].

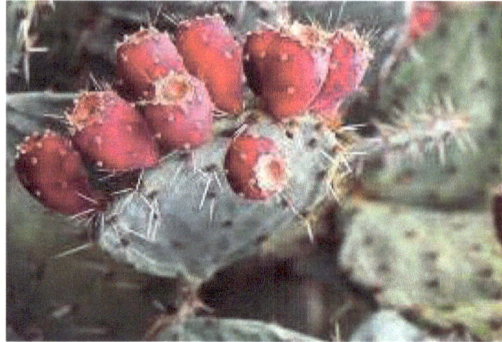

Fig. 5. *Cactus pear.*

Prickly pear fruit (Fig. **6**), like cactus pear fruit, has long been used in traditional medicine to treat a variety of ailments, including ulcers, dyspnea, and glaucoma, as well as liver illnesses, wounds, and tiredness [45, 46]. Antioxidant properties have been proven in European and Asian prickly pear cultivars, with significant reductions in OS in patients and prevention of chronic diseases [72]. In human and animal models, certain preparations of the fleshy stems (cladodes) have been evaluated for the management of diabetic symptomatology [73]. Fresh stems and prickly pear are also great sources of fibre, according to some writers, and these components help lower blood sugar and cholesterol levels in the plasma [74]. The bioactive substances in the prickly pear fruit, such as vitamin C and vitamin E, polyphenols, carotenoids, flavonoid compounds (for example, kaempherol, quercetin, and isorhamnetin), taurine, and pigments, have been attributed to the fruit's functional food status [45, 52 - 57].

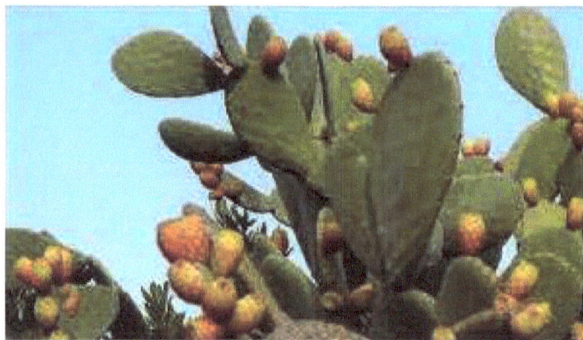

Fig. 6. *Cactus pear fruit.*

Chamomile (*Matricaria Chamomilla or Chamomilla Recutita*)

While there is a large body of evidence supporting the health advantages of drinking teas made from *Camilla sinensis* (*i.e.*, black and green teas) [63], verification-based data on the effects of high consumption of herbal teas, or tisanes, is limited. Chamomile [75] is one of the most popular single-ingredient herbal beverages. Chamomile (*Matricaria chamomilla* or *Chamomilla recutita*) is a plant of the Asteraceae family that is native to Europe and is found all over the world, save in tropical and polar climates. This plant has been used for its remedial properties since the ancient Egyptian and Greek civilizations, and it presently is regularly used as an antiseptic, antiphlogistic, diuretic, expectorant, febrifuge, sedative, anti-inflammatory, and anticarcinogenic [18] (Fig. **7**).

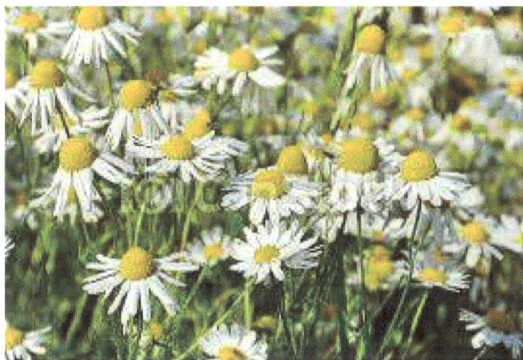

Fig. 7. *Chamomilla recutita.*

The anti-inflammatory capability and moderating effects of Hsp on apigenin and quercetin flavonoids, as well as the anti-inflammatory, antioxidant, and antiseptic properties identified in -bisabolol, guargazulene, and chamazulene [18, 65, 66], have all been documented. Bisabolol, chamazulene, cyclic sesquiterpenes, bisabolol oxides, and other azulenes and terpenes make up the essential oil derived from the chamomile flower, which varies from 0.42 percent to 2 percent [76].

Silymarin (*Silybum marianum*)

The scientific name for milk thistle (Mt) or St. Mary's thistle is *Silybum marianum* (Fig. **8**). It is a Mediterranean plant of the Asteraceae family that grows in the Mediterranean area. It has thorny branches, milky sap, and oval leaves that may grow up to 30 cm in length; its blooms are brilliant pink and up to 8 cm in diameter [77 - 80]. Milk thistle (Mt) grows wild in southern Europe, North Africa, and the Middle East, although it is cultivated in Hungary, China, and nations in South America, including Argentina, Venezuela, and Ecuador. It has been used as a dietary supplement in Mexico for many years [18, 75]. In the 1960s, German scientists conducted a chemical investigation of the milk thistle fruit, isolating a crude extract made up of strong chemicals with hepatoprotective properties, which they dubbed silymarin. Silybin A, silybin B, isosilybin A, isosilybin B, silychristine A, silychristine B, and silydianine were discovered to be the major constituents of silymarin in 1975 [18, 76]. Flavonolignans, or a combination of flavonoids and lignin structures, are now thought to be the chemical components of silymarin [18, 81]. It is one of the most studied plant extracts, having recognised mechanisms of action for the treatment of toxic liver damage when taken orally. Silymarin has been used as a defensive treatment in acute and chronic liver diseases [18, 81].

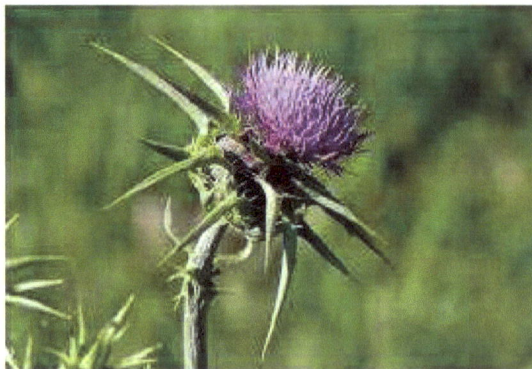

Fig. 8. *Silybum marianum.*

Its anti-toxin properties are linked to a variety of processes, including limiting toxin dissemination into hepatocytes, boosting SOD activity, raising glutathione tissue levels, preventing lipid peroxidation, and promoting hepatocyte protein synthesis. Because of the phenolic character of its flavonolignans, silymarin's hepatoprotective action can be explained by its antioxidant capabilities. It also prevents hepatotoxic substances from entering hepatocytes by stimulating liver cell regeneration and cell membrane stability [18, 79]. Silymarin has also been advantageous in dropping the chances for developing certain Cancers [18, 82].

Trigonella-foecum-graecum

Trigonella (methi in Hindi, fenugreek in English) is a member of the Fabaceae family. It is an annual plant that is widely cultivated in India, Pakistan, Egypt, and the Middle East [12] (Fig. **9**). *Trigonella* has grown in popularity as a result of its pungent odour and therapeutic capabilities for treating a variety of ailments [83]. *Trigonella* leaf is high in calcium, iron, beta-carotene, and other phytonutrients. Culinary dishes are made using leaves and seeds [14]. Flavonoids, polysaccharides, saponins, fibres, and alkaloids such as trigocoumarin, choline, and trigonelline are the primary chemical ingredients of *Trigonella* [15]. *Trigonella* leaf extracts have been found to have cytoprotective, antioxidant, and hepatoprotective properties, suggesting that they might be used as a dietary supplement or in liver disease formulations. Increased levels of LPO and GSH, as well as reduced antioxidant activity such as SOD, GST, and catalase, indicate that DM causes oxidative stress in the rat liver. Trigonella's disclosure resulted in a significant recovery in skewed values of these metrics. On the basis of the above information, it is possible to conclude that natural *Trigonella* has antioxidative and antilipidemic capabilities. It's also helpful in cases of pesticide-induced hepatotoxicity.

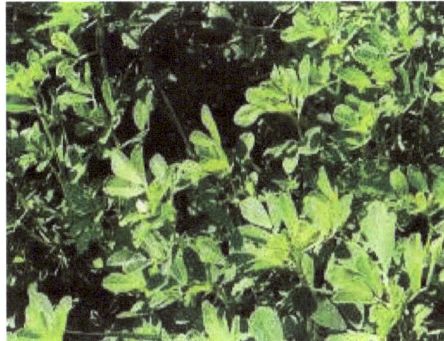

Fig. 9. *Trigonella-foecum-graecum.*

Trigonella may have antiulcer, wound-healing, CNS stimulant, immunomodulatory, antioxidant, antidiabetic, antineoplastic, anti-inflammatory, and antipyretic activities. The extracts from the dried seeds of *Trigonella* show hepatoprotective action in a rat model of thioacetamide-induced liver cirrhosis [84-85]. *Trigonella* methanol extract has a significant hepatoprotective effect against CCl4-induced hepatotoxicity [80].

Allium cepa

The garden onion, *Allium cepa* (Fig. **10**), belongs to the Liliaceae family. It is widely grown in China, India, and the United States. It has a high carbohydrate, potassium, sodium, and phosphorus content. It's been used for centuries to treat intestinal infections, earaches, eye infections, migraines, sleepiness, urinary tract infections, burning ulcers, and coughs [81]. Antiviral, antifungal, antibacterial, and antiparasitic properties, as well as antihypertensive, hypoglycemic, antithrombotic, antihyperlipidemic, anti-inflammatory, and antioxidant properties [21 - 23]. In adult male albino Wistar rats, aqueous bulb extract of *A. cepa* has hepatoprotective and hepatotoxic properties [82].

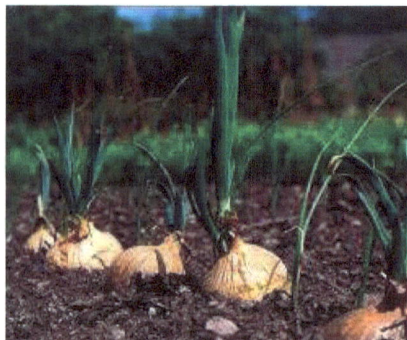

Fig. 10. *Allium cepa.*

Azadiracta indica

Azadiracta indica, often known as Nimba or Neem, is a common tree in India (Fig. **11**). It is a member of the Meliaceae family and is commonly referred to as neem. A. indica is a tropical plant native to India and Burma, where it thrives in humid and semi-humid climates. It is a fast-growing tree that may reach a height of 15-20 metres, with a chance of reaching 35-40 metres. Leprosy, intestinal worms, skin infections, constipation, epistaxis, biliary ailment, anorexia, blood morbidity, and biliousness have all been documented to benefit from A. indica. Bitter active components are found in several areas of the plant [83]. It reduced blood glucose levels and slowed the development of stomach ulcers [84]. Researchers discovered that aqueous, alcoholic, ethyl acetate and petroleum ether extracts of A. indica leaves have hepatoprotective properties. The antioxidant and hepatoprotective activity of juice extracted from the young stem bark of *A. indica* was also tested against CCl4-induced liver injury [85]. The findings suggested that the antioxidant and hepatoprotective effects of fresh neem juice are most likely due to its free radical scavenging activity.

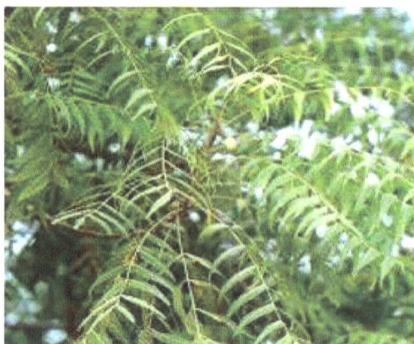

Fig. 11. *Azadiracta indica.*

Boerhavia diffusa

Because of their protection and efficiency, the roots of *Boerhavia diffusa* (Punarnava) are used to treat a variety of liver ailments (Fig. **12**). Punarnava is a Sanskrit term that means "body renewer." Purarnava has long been regarded as one of the most important medicinal plants in India. In India, South America, and Africa, *B. diffusa* (family Nyctaginaceae) is an important medicinal herb for treating liver problems. Different portions of the plant, notably the roots, have been utilised to treat gastrointestinal, hepatoprotective, and gynaecological problems, as well as immunomodulation, antifibrinolytics, anticancer action, antidiabetic activity, anti-inflammation, and diuresis. The phytochemical ingredients and therapeutic actions of *B. diffusa* have been widely credited. Isoflavonoids (rotenoids), flavonoids, flavonoid glycosides, xanthenes, purine nucleosides, lignans, ecdysteroids, and steroids are among the substances found in the roots [33]. B. diffusa is useful for treating paracetamol and acetaminophen-induced hepatotoxicity [34 - 37]. Punarnava has also been shown to be useful in the treatment of jaundice [38, 39]. *B. diffusa's* hepatoprotective benefits may be due to its oxidant property, membrane stabilising activity, or capacity to maintain near-normal levels of free radical enzymes and GSH, all of which protect the liver.

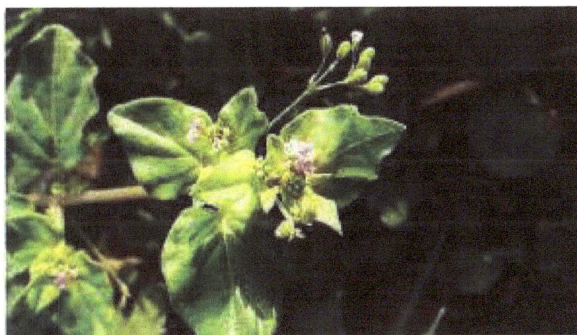

Fig. 12. *Boerhavia diffusa.*

Curcuma longa

Curcuma longa, also known as turmeric (Haridra or Haldi in Hindi), is a perennial rhizomatous plant (Fig. **13**). It is a member of the Zingiberaceae family and is endemic to South Asia. It's a well-liked component for a variety of meals. Turmeric has also been used in traditional medicine, and it has been shown to be effective in the treatment of jaundice and other liver illnesses, parasite infections, ulcers, and many skin ailments. *C. longa* rhizome juice can be used to treat a variety of ailments, including anthelmintics, asthma, gonorrhea, and urinary infections. Its essential oil is also utilised for carminative, stomachic, and tonic purposes [41, 42]. In conventional medicine, a number of herbal remedies have been used to treat liver disorders, together with liver cirrhosis [43, 44]. Different extracts of *C. longa* are reported to have hepatoprotective activity alongside CCl_4 and TAA-induced toxicity [42 - 45].

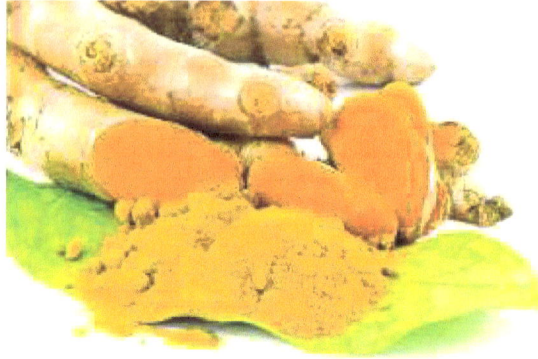

Fig. 13. *Curcuma longa.*

Ocimum Sanctum

It provides a wide variety of possible benefits. Tulsi is the common name for Ocimum sanctum (family Lamiaceae). O. sanctum is a popular Ayurvedic treatment for the common cold, headaches, stomach problems, inflammation, heart illness, various poisonings, and malaria [46] (Fig. **14**). The therapeutic effects of many components of this plant have been recorded. Various researchers have found that this plant has anabolic, hypotensive, cardiac depressive, smooth muscle relaxant, antifertility, and anti-stress characteristics [47]. Several researchers have indicated that O. sanctum has hepatotoxic potential against paracetamol, CCl4, and lead-induced liver injury [11, 46, 48 - 51].

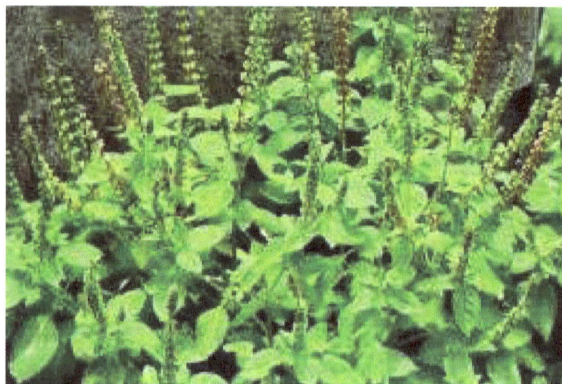

Fig. 14. Ocimum sanctum

Table 1. Hepatoprotective activity of the medicinal plants

Name of the Plant	Source or Family	Plant parts used	Hepatotoxicity inducing agents	Extracts studied	Biochemical and Histopathological Parameters studied
Orthosiphon stamineus	Lamiaceae	Leaves	Acetaminophen	Methanol extract	AST, ALT, and ALP
Baliospermum montanum	Euphorbiaceae	Roots	Paracetamol	Alcohol, chloroform extract	SGPT, SGOT, and alkaline phosphate,
Tridax procumbens	Asteraceae	Leaves	Carbon tetrachloride	Ethanolic extract	Glutathione, superoxide dismutase, and catalase
Glycyrrhiza glabra Linn	Fabaceae	Root powder	Carbon tetrachloride	Root powder mixed with animal feed	TBARS, CD, SOD, CAT, GST, GSH-Px, GSH, Lipid Peroxidation
Phyllanthus niruri 1	Euphorbiaceae	Leaves and fruits	Carbon tetrachloride	Methanolic and aqueous	glutamate oxaloacetate transaminase (GOT) and glutamate pyruvate
Cochlospermum Planchoni 11	Coclospermaceae	Rhizomes	Carbon tetrachloride	Aqueous	Total bilirubin Alkaline phosphatase Alanine aminotransferase
Saururus chinensis 12	Saururaceae	Whole plant	Carbon tetrachloride	Ethanol	Alanine aminotransferase (ALT), aspartate aminotransferase (AST), hyaluronic acid (HA), hepatic malondialdehyde (MDA) content
'Teng-Khia-U' 13 derived from the entire plants of *Elephantopus scaber L., E. mollis H.B.K.,* and *Pseudoelephantopus spicatus* (Juss.) Rohr	Asteraceae	Whole plant	D-galactosamine (d-gain)- and acetaminophen (apap)	Aqueous	serum glutamate-oxalat--transaminase (sGOT) and the serum glutamate pyruvate-transaminase (sGPT)
Fructus Schisandrae chinensis (LFS) with *Astragalus polysaccharides (APS)*	Magnoliaceae	Dried fructus	Carbon tetrachloride	Ethanol	Alanine aminotransferase (ALT), aspartate aminotransferase (AST), alkaline phosphatase (ALP) malondialdehyde (MDA)
Cordia macleodii	Boraginaceae	Leaves	Carbon tetrachloride	Ethanolic	Glutamate pyruvate transaminase (GPT), serum glutamate oxaloacetate transaminase (GOT)

(Table 1) cont.....

Name of the Plant	Source or Family	Plant parts used	Hepatotoxicity inducing agents	Extracts studied	Biochemical and Histopathological Parameters studied
Arachniodes exilis	Dryopteridaceae	Rhizomes	Carbon tetrachloride	Ethanol	Lipid peroxide, DPPH, ABTS, superoxide anion, hydroxyl radical and hydrogen peroxide
Momordica dioica 1	Cucurbitaceae	Leaves	Carbon tetrachloride	Ethanolic and aqueous	Serum glutamate oxaloacetate transaminase (AST), Serum glutamate pyruvate transaminase (ALT),

CONCLUSION

Drug and chemical-induced hepatotoxicity is the most frequent iatrogenic condition. Changeable degrees of fibrosis, cirrhosis, or neoplasia define the chronic liver disease. According to a WHO estimate, nearly 80% of the world's population accepts herbal medications for their basic healthcare requirements in developing nations. Even from medications, modern medicine offers a fairly limited selection of treatments and therapies for liver fortification. Thus, the use of herbal treatments, which are easy to get and much easier to prepare formulations for the management of any type of hepatotoxicity, is gaining favour across the world. These medicines are fortunately highly efficient and cost-effective, prompting researchers to continue their hunt for better drugs, more strong plant-active ingredients, and more pleasant formulations. In this chapter, every effort has been made to gather and consolidate information on a few hepatoprotective plants that will be valuable to society as it moves into the realm of alternative medicine.

REFERENCES

[1]   Lin, J.H.; Lu, A.Y. Role of pharmacokinetics and metabolism in drug discovery and development. *Pharmacol. Rev.,* **1997**, *49*(4), 403-449.
[PMID: 9443165]

[2]   Shanani, S. Evaluation of hepatoprotective efficacy of APCL- A polyherbal formulation *in vivo* in rats. *Indian Drugs,* **1999**, *36*, 628-631.

[3]   Subramoniam, A.; Pushpangadan, P. Development of phytomedicine for liver diseases. *Indian J. Pharmacol.,* **1999**, *31*, 166-175.

[4]   Adewusi, E.A.; Afolayan, A.J. A review of natural products with hepatoprotective activity. *J. Med. Plants Res.,* **2010**, *4*, 1318-1334.

[5]   Ahsan, M.R.; Islam, K.M.; Bulbul, I.J. Hepatoprotective activity of Methanol Extract of some medicinal plants against carbon tetrachloride-induced hepatotoxicity in rats. *Glob. J. Pharmacol.,* **2009**, *3*, 116-122.

[6]   Asha, V.V.; Pushpangadan, P. Preliminary evaluation of the anti-hepatotoxic activity of *Phyllanthus kozhikodianus, Phyllanthus maderspatensis* and *Solanum indicum. Fitoterapia,* **1998**, *59*, 255-259.

[7]   Casafont-Morencos, F.; Puente, A.; Pons-Romero, F. Infecciones bacterianas y parasitarias del hígado.

Medicine, **2008**, *10*, 563-569.

[8]   Amengual-Guedan, M.J.; Rodríguez Sánchez, J.L. Autoinmunidad en las enfermedades del hígado (I). *Inmunologia,* **2000**, *19*, 90-102.

[9]   Deshwal, N.; Sharma, A.K.; Sharma, P. Review on hepatoprotective plants. *Int. J. Pharm. Sci. Rev. Res.,* **2011**, *7*, 15-26.

[10]   Chattopadhyay, R.R. Possible mechanism of hepatoprotective activity of *Azadirachta indica* leaf extract: Part II. *J. Ethnopharmacol.,* **2003**, *89*(2-3), 217-219.
        [http://dx.doi.org/10.1016/j.jep.2003.08.006] [PMID: 14611885]

[11]   Gupta, S.S. Prospects and perspectives of natural plant products in medicine. *Indian J. Pharmacol.,* **1994**, *26*, 1-12.

[12]   Kasdallah-Grissa, A.; Mornagui, B.; Aouani, E.; Hammami, M.; Gharbi, N.; Kamoun, A.; El-Fazaa, S. Protective effect of resveratrol on ethanol-induced lipid peroxidation in rats. *Alcohol Alcohol.,* **2006**, *41*(3), 236-239.
        [http://dx.doi.org/10.1093/alcalc/agh256] [PMID: 16517551]

[13]   Sumaya-Martínez, M.T.; Cruz-Jaime, S.; Madrigal-Santillán, E.; García-Paredes, J.D.; Cariño-Cortés, R.; Cruz-Cansino, N.; Valadez-Vega, C.; Martinez-Cardenas, L.; Alanís-García, E. Betalain, acid ascorbic, phenolic contents and antioxidant properties of purple, red, yellow and white cactus pears. *Int. J. Mol. Sci.,* **2011**, *12*(10), 6452-6468.
        [http://dx.doi.org/10.3390/ijms12106452] [PMID: 22072899]

[14]   Madrigal-Santillán, E.; Fragoso-Antonio, S.; Valadez-Vega, C.; Solano-Solano, G.; Pérez, C.Z.; Sánchez-Gutiérrez, M.; Izquierdo-Vega, J.A.; Gutiérrez-Salinas, J.; Esquivel-Soto, J.; Esquivel-Chirino, C.; Sumaya-Martínez, T.; Fregoso-Aguilar, T.; Mendoza-Pérez, J.; Morales-González, J.A. Investigation on the protective effects of cranberry against the DNA damage induced by benzo[a]pyrene. *Molecules,* **2012**, *17*(4), 4435-4451.
        [http://dx.doi.org/10.3390/molecules17044435] [PMID: 22499190]

[15]   Olaleye, M.T.; Adegboye, O.O.; Akindahunsi, A.A. *Alchornea cordifolia* extract protects wistar albino rats against acetaminophen inducedliver damage. *Afr. J. Biotechnol.,* **2006**, *5*, 2439-2445.

[16]   Bhawna, S.; Kumar, S.U. Hepatoprotective activity of some indigenous plants. *Int. J. Pharm. Tech. Res.,* **2009**, *4*, 1330-1334.

[17]   Gupta, V.; Kohli, K.; Ghaiye, P.; Bansal, P.; Lather, A. Pharmacological potentials of citrus paradise-An overview. *Int. J. Physiother. Res.,* **2011**, *1*, 8-17.

[18]   Madrigal, S.E.; Madrigal, B.E.; Cruz, J.S.; Valadez, V.M.C.; Sumaya, M.M.T.; Pérez, Á.K.G.; Morales, G.J.A. The chemoprevention of chronic degenerative disease through dietary antioxidants: Progress, promise and evidences. In: *Oxidative stress and chronic degenerative diseases-a role for antioxidants*; Morales-González, J.A., Ed.; Croatia InTech: Rijeka, **2013**; pp. 155-185.
        [http://dx.doi.org/10.5772/52162]

[19]   Monroe, K.R.; Murphy, S.P.; Kolonel, L.N.; Pike, M.C. Prospective study of grapefruit intake and risk of breast cancer in postmenopausal women: The multiethnic cohort study. *Br. J. Cancer,* **2007**, *97*(3), 440-445.
        [http://dx.doi.org/10.1038/sj.bjc.6603880] [PMID: 17622247]

[20]   Kumar, A.; Dogra, S.; Prakash, A. Protective effect of naringin, a citrus flavonoid, against colchicine-induced cognitive dysfunction and oxidative damage in rats. *J. Med. Food,* **2010**, *13*(4), 976-984.
        [http://dx.doi.org/10.1089/jmf.2009.1251] [PMID: 20673063]

[21]   Pereira, R.; Andrades, N.; Paulino, N.; Sawaya, A.; Eberlin, M.; Marcucci, M.; Favero, G.; Novak, E.; Bydlowski, S. Synthesis and characterization of a metal complex containing naringin and Cu, and its antioxidant, antimicrobial, antiinflammatory and tumor cell cytotoxicity. *Molecules,* **2007**, *12*(7), 1352-1366.
        [http://dx.doi.org/10.3390/12071352] [PMID: 17909491]

[22] Parmar, N.S. The gastric anti-ulcer activity of naringenin, a specific histidine decarboxylase inhibitor. *Int. J. Tissue React.,* **1983**, *5*(4), 415-420.
[PMID: 6671888]

[23] Lee, M.H.; Yoon, S.; Moon, J.O. The flavonoid naringenin inhibits dimethylnitrosamine-induced liver damage in rats. *Biol. Pharm. Bull.,* **2004**, *27*(1), 72-76.
[http://dx.doi.org/10.1248/bpb.27.72] [PMID: 14709902]

[24] Jayaraman, J.; Veerappan, M.; Namasivayam, N. Potential beneficial effect of naringenin on lipid peroxidation and antioxidant status in rats with ethanol-induced hepatotoxicity. *J. Pharm. Pharmacol.,* **2010**, *61*(10), 1383-1390.
[http://dx.doi.org/10.1211/jpp.61.10.0016] [PMID: 19814872]

[25] Jayaraman, J.; Namasivayam, N. Naringenin modulates circulatory lipid peroxidation, anti-oxidant status and hepatic alcohol metabolizing enzymes in rats with ethanol induced liver injury. *Fundam. Clin. Pharmacol.,* **2011**, *25*(6), 682-689.
[http://dx.doi.org/10.1111/j.1472-8206.2010.00899.x] [PMID: 21105911]

[26] Seo, H.J.; Jeong, K.S.; Lee, M.K.; Park, Y.B.; Jung, U.J.; Kim, H.J.; Choi, M.S. Role of naringin supplement in regulation of lipid and ethanol metabolism in rats. *Life Sci.,* **2003**, *73*(7), 933-946.
[http://dx.doi.org/10.1016/S0024-3205(03)00358-8] [PMID: 12798418]

[27] Seeram, N.P. Berry fruits: Compositional elements, biochemical activities, and the impact of their intake on human health, performance, and disease. *J. Agric. Food Chem.,* **2008**, *56*(3), 627-629.
[http://dx.doi.org/10.1021/jf071988k] [PMID: 18211023]

[28] Neto, C.C. Cranberry and its phytochemicals: A review of *in vitro* anticancer studies. *J. Nutr.,* **2007**, *137*(1), 186S-193S.
[http://dx.doi.org/10.1093/jn/137.1.186S] [PMID: 17182824]

[29] Cederbaum, A.I.; Lu, Y.; Wu, D. Role of oxidative stress in alcohol-induced liver injury. *Arch. Toxicol.,* **2009**, *83*(6), 519-548.
[http://dx.doi.org/10.1007/s00204-009-0432-0] [PMID: 19448996]

[30] Ade, N.; Leon, F.; Pallardy, M.; Peiffer, J.L.; Kerdine-Romer, S.; Tissier, M.H.; Bonnet, P.A.; Fabre, I.; Ourlin, J.C. HMOX1 and NQO1 genes are upregulated in response to contact sensitizers in dendritic cells and THP-1 cell line: role of the Keap1/Nrf2 pathway. *Toxicol. Sci.,* **2009**, *107*(2), 451-460.
[http://dx.doi.org/10.1093/toxsci/kfn243] [PMID: 19033392]

[31] Surh, Y.J.; Kundu, J.; Na, H.K. Nrf2 as a master redox switch in turning on the cellular signaling involved in the induction of cytoprotective genes by some chemopreventive phytochemicals. *Planta Med.,* **2008**, *74*(13), 1526-1539.
[http://dx.doi.org/10.1055/s-0028-1088302] [PMID: 18937164]

[32] Wang, Y.P.; Cheng, M.L.; Zhang, B.F.; Mu, M.; Zhou, M.Y.; Wu, J.; Li, C.X. Effect of blueberry on hepatic and immunological functions in mice. *Hepatobiliary Pancreat. Dis. Int.,* **2010**, *9*(2), 164-168.
[PMID: 20382588]

[33] Cheshchevik, V.T.; Lapshina, E.A.; Dremza, I.K.; Zabrodskaya, S.V.; Reiter, R.J.; Prokopchik, N.I.; Zavodnik, I.B. Rat liver mitochondrial damage under acute or chronic carbon tetrachloride-induced intoxication: Protection by melatonin and cranberry flavonoids. *Toxicol. Appl. Pharmacol.,* **2012**, *261*(3), 271-279.
[http://dx.doi.org/10.1016/j.taap.2012.04.007] [PMID: 22521486]

[34] Shin, M.O.; Yoon, S.; Moon, J.O. The proanthocyanidins inhibit dimethylnitrosamine-induced liver damage in rats. *Arch. Pharm. Res.,* **2010**, *33*(1), 167-173.
[http://dx.doi.org/10.1007/s12272-010-2239-1] [PMID: 20191358]

[35] Arroyo-García, R.; Ruiz-García, L.; Bolling, L.; Ocete, R.; López, M.A.; Arnold, C.; Ergul, A.; Söylemezo"lu, G.; Uzun, H.I.; Cabello, F.; Ibáñez, J.; Aradhya, M.K.; Atanassov, A.; Atanassov, I.;

Balint, S.; Cenis, J.L.; Costantini, L.; Gorislavets, S.; Grando, M.S.; Klein, B.Y.; McGOVERN, P.E.; Merdinoglu, D.; Pejic, I.; Pelsy, F.; Primikirios, N.; Risovannaya, V.; Roubelakis-Angelakis, K.A.; Snoussi, H.; Sotiri, P.; Tamhankar, S.; This, P.; Troshin, L.; Malpica, J.M.; Lefort, F.; Martinez-Zapater, J.M. Multiple origins of cultivated grapevine (*Vitis vinifera* L. ssp. sativa) based on chloroplast DNA polymorphisms. *Mol. Ecol.,* **2006**, *15*(12), 3707-3714.
[http://dx.doi.org/10.1111/j.1365-294X.2006.03049.x] [PMID: 17032268]

[36] Šuklje, K.; Lisjak, K.; Baša Česnik, H.; Janeš, L.; Du Toit, W.; Coetzee, Z.; Vanzo, A.; Deloire, A. Classification of grape berries according to diameter and total soluble solids to study the effect of light and temperature on methoxypyrazine, glutathione, and hydroxycinnamate evolution during ripening of Sauvignon blanc (*Vitis vinifera* L.). *J. Agric. Food Chem.,* **2012**, *60*(37), 9454-9461.
[http://dx.doi.org/10.1021/jf3020766] [PMID: 22946638]

[37] Hernández-Jiménez, A.; Gil-Muñoz, R.; Ruiz-García, Y.; López-Roca, J.M.; Martinez-Cutillas, A.; Gómez-Plaza, E. Evaluating the polyphenol profile in three segregating grape (*Vitis vinifera* L.) populations. *J. Anal. Methods Chem.,* **2013**, *2013*, 1-9.
[http://dx.doi.org/10.1155/2013/572896] [PMID: 23986879]

[38] De Nisco, M.; Manfra, M.; Bolognese, A.; Sofo, A.; Scopa, A.; Tenore, G.C.; Pagano, F.; Milite, C.; Russo, M.T. Nutraceutical properties and polyphenolic profile of berry skin and wine of Vitis vinifera L. (cv. Aglianico). *Food Chem.,* **2013**, *140*(4), 623-629.
[http://dx.doi.org/10.1016/j.foodchem.2012.10.123] [PMID: 23692745]

[39] Sandoval, M.; Lazarte, K.; Arnao, I. Hepatoprotección antioxidante de la cáscara y semilla de Vitis vinifera L. (uva). *An. Fac. Med., Univ. Nac. Mayor San Marcos,* **2013**, *69*(4), 250-259.
[http://dx.doi.org/10.15381/anales.v69i4.1125]

[40] Katalinic, V.; Mozina, S.S.; Generalic, I.; Skroza, D.; Ljubenkov, I.; Klancnik, A. Phenolic profile, antioxidant capacity, and antimicrobial activity of leaf extracts from six *Vitis vinifera* L. Varieties. *Int. J. Food Prop.,* **2013**, *16*(1), 45-60.
[http://dx.doi.org/10.1080/10942912.2010.526274]

[41] Dani, C.; Oliboni, L.S.; Pasquali, M.A.B.; Oliveira, M.R.; Umezu, F.M.; Salvador, M.; Moreira, J.C.F.; Henriques, J.A.P. Intake of purple grape juice as a hepatoprotective agent in Wistar rats. *J. Med. Food,* **2008**, *11*(1), 127-132.
[http://dx.doi.org/10.1089/jmf.2007.558] [PMID: 18361748]

[42] Dogan, A.; Celik, I. Hepatoprotective and antioxidant activities of grapeseeds against ethanol-induced oxidative stress in rats. *Br. J. Nutr.,* **2012**, *107*(1), 45-51.
[http://dx.doi.org/10.1017/S0007114511002650] [PMID: 21733325]

[43] Kasdallah-Grissa, A.; Mornagui, B.; Aouani, E.; Hammami, M.; El May, M.; Gharbi, N.; Kamoun, A.; El-Fazaâ, S. Resveratrol, a red wine polyphenol, attenuates ethanol-induced oxidative stress in rat liver. *Life Sci.,* **2007**, *80*(11), 1033-1039.
[http://dx.doi.org/10.1016/j.lfs.2006.11.044] [PMID: 17258234]

[44] Gurocak, S.; Karabulut, E.; Karadag, N.; Ozgor, D.; Ozkeles, N.; Karabulut, A.B. Preventive effects of resveratrol against azoxymethane induced damage in rat liver. *Asian Pac. J. Cancer Prev.,* **2013**, *14*(4), 2367-2370.
[http://dx.doi.org/10.7314/APJCP.2013.14.4.2367] [PMID: 23725142]

[45] Madrigal-Santillán, E.; García-Melo, F.; Morales-González, J.; Vázquez-Alvarado, P.; Muñoz-Juárez, S.; Zuñiga-Pérez, C.; Sumaya-Martínez, M.; Madrigal-Bujaidar, E.; Hernández-Ceruelos, A. Antioxidant and anticlastogenic capacity of prickly pear juice. *Nutrients,* **2013**, *5*(10), 4145-4158.
[http://dx.doi.org/10.3390/nu5104145] [PMID: 24145870]

[46] Kaur, M.; Kaur, A.; Sharma, R. Pharmacological actions of *Opuntia ficus indica:* A Review. *J. Appl. Pharm. Sci.,* **2012**, *2*, 15-18.
[http://dx.doi.org/10.7324/JAPS.2012.2703]

[47] Livrea, M.A.; Tesoriere, L. Antioxidant activities of prickly pear (*opuntia ficus indica*) fruit and its.

betalains, betanin and indicaxanthin. In: *Herbal and Traditional Medicine. Molecular Aspects of Health*; Packer, L.; Nam, O.C.; Halliwell, B., Eds.; Marcel Dekker: New York, **2004**; pp. 537-556.
[http://dx.doi.org/10.1201/9780203025901.ch24]

[48]   Ibañez-Camacho, R.; Meckes-Lozoya, M.; Mellado-Campos, V. The hypoglucemic effect of *opuntia streptacantha* studied in different animal experimental models. *J. Ethnopharmacol.*, **1983**, *7*(2), 175-181.
[http://dx.doi.org/10.1016/0378-8741(83)90019-3] [PMID: 6865450]

[49]   Trejo-González, A.; Gabriel-Ortiz, G.; Puebla-Pérez, A.M.; Huízar-Contreras, M.D.; del Rosario Munguía-Mazariegos, M.; Mejía-Arreguín, S.; Calva, E. A purified extract from prickly pear cactus (*Opuntia fuliginosa*) controls experimentally induced diabetes in rats. *J. Ethnopharmacol.*, **1996**, *55*(1), 27-33.
[http://dx.doi.org/10.1016/S0378-8741(96)01467-5] [PMID: 9121164]

[50]   Fernandez, M.L.; Lin, E.C.K.; Trejo, A.; McNamara, D.J. Prickly pear (Opuntia sp.) pectin reverses low density lipoprotein receptor suppression induced by a hypercholesterolemic diet in guinea pigs. *J. Nutr.*, **1992**, *122*(12), 2330-2340.
[http://dx.doi.org/10.1093/jn/122.12.2330] [PMID: 1333520]

[51]   Muñoz de Chávez, M.; Chávez, A.; Valles, V.; Roldán, J.A. The nopal: A plant of manifold qualities. *World Rev. Nutr. Diet.*, **1995**, *77*, 109-134.
[http://dx.doi.org/10.1159/000424468] [PMID: 7732696]

[52]   Sawaya, W.N.; Khatchadourian, H.A.; Safi, W.M.; Al-Muhammad, H.M. Chemical characterization of prickly pear pulp, *Opuntia ficus-indica*, and the manufacturing of prickly pear jam. *Int. J. Food Sci. Technol.*, **1983**, *18*(2), 183-193.
[http://dx.doi.org/10.1111/j.1365-2621.1983.tb00259.x]

[53]   Kuti, J.O. Antioxidant compounds from four opuntia cactus pear fruit varieties. *Food Chem.*, **2004**, *85*(4), 527-533.
[http://dx.doi.org/10.1016/S0308-8146(03)00184-5]

[54]   Fernández-López, J.A.; Almela, L.; Obón, J.M.; Castellar, R. Determination of antioxidant constituents in cactus pear fruits. *Plant Foods Hum. Nutr.*, **2010**, *65*(3), 253-259.
[http://dx.doi.org/10.1007/s11130-010-0189-x] [PMID: 20811778]

[55]   Castellar, R.; Obón, J.M.; Alacid, M.; Fernández-López, J.A. Color properties and stability of betacyanins from Opuntia fruits. *J. Agric. Food Chem.*, **2003**, *51*(9), 2772-2776.
[http://dx.doi.org/10.1021/jf021045h] [PMID: 12696971]

[56]   Livrea, M.A.; Tesoriere, L. Antioxidative effects of cactus pear [*Opuntia ficus indica* (L) Mill] fruits from Sicily and bioavailability of betalain components in healthy humans. *Acta Hortic.*, **2009**, *811*(811), 197-204.
[http://dx.doi.org/10.17660/ActaHortic.2009.811.24]

[57]   Piga, A. Cactus Pear: A fruit of nutraceutical and functional cactus pear: A fruit of nutraceutical and functional. *J. Prof. Assoc. Cactus Dev.*, **2004**, *6*, 9-22.

[58]   Wiese, J.; McPherson, S.; Odden, M.C.; Shlipak, M.G. Effect of *Opuntia ficus indica* on symptoms of the alcohol hangover. *Arch. Intern. Med.*, **2004**, *164*(12), 1334-1340.
[http://dx.doi.org/10.1001/archinte.164.12.1334] [PMID: 15226168]

[59]   Ncibi, S.; Ben Othman, M.; Akacha, A.; Krifi, M.N.; Zourgui, L. Opuntia ficus indica extract protects against chlorpyrifos-induced damage on mice liver. *Food Chem. Toxicol.*, **2008**, *46*(2), 797-802.
[http://dx.doi.org/10.1016/j.fct.2007.08.047] [PMID: 17980473]

[60]   Brahmi, D.; Ayed, Y.; Bouaziz, C.; Zourgui, L.; Hassen, W.; Bacha, H. Hepatoprotective effect of cactus extract against carcinogenicity of benzo(a)pyrene on liver of Balb/C mice. *J. Med. Plants Res.*, **2011**, *5*, 4627-4639.

[61]   Brahmi, D.; Bouaziz, C.; Ayed, Y.; Ben Mansour, H.; Zourgui, L.; Bacha, H. Chemopreventive effect

of cactus *Opuntia ficus indica* on oxidative stress and genotoxicity of aflatoxin B1. *Nutr. Metab.,* **2011**, *8*(1), 73.
[http://dx.doi.org/10.1186/1743-7075-8-73] [PMID: 22008149]

[62] Alimi, H.; Hfaeidh, N.; Mbarki, S.; Bouoni, Z.; Sakly, M.; Rouma, K.B. Evaluation of *Opuntia ficus indica f. inermis* fruit juice hepatoprotective effect upon ethanol toxicity in rats. *Gen. Physiol. Biophys.,* **2012**, *31*(3), 335-342.
[http://dx.doi.org/10.4149/gpb_2012_038] [PMID: 23047946]

[63] McKay, D.L.; Blumberg, J.B. The role of tea in human health: An update. *J. Am. Coll. Nutr.,* **2002**, *21*(1), 1-13.
[http://dx.doi.org/10.1080/07315724.2002.10719187] [PMID: 11838881]

[64] McKay, D.L.; Blumberg, J.B. A Review of the bioactivity and potential health benefits of chamomile tea (Matricaria recutita L.). *Phytother. Res.,* **2006**, *20*(7), 519-530.
[http://dx.doi.org/10.1002/ptr.1900] [PMID: 16628544]

[65] Jakolev, V.; Issac, O.; Flaskamp, E. Pharmacological investigation with compounds of chamazulene and matricine. *Planta Med.,* **1983**, *49*, 67-73.

[66] Viola, H.; Wasowski, C.; Levi de Stein, M.; Wolfman, C.; Silveira, R.; Dajas, F.; Medina, J.; Paladini, A. Apigenin, a component of matricaria recutita flowers, is a central benzodiazepine receptors-ligand with anxiolytic effects. *Planta Med.,* **1995**, *61*(3), 213-216.
[http://dx.doi.org/10.1055/s-2006-958058] [PMID: 7617761]

[67] McKay, D.L.; Blumberg, J.B. A review of the bioactivity and potential health benefits of peppermint tea (Mentha piperita L.). *Phytother. Res.,* **2006**, *20*(8), 619-633.
[http://dx.doi.org/10.1002/ptr.1936] [PMID: 16767798]

[68] Hernández-Ceruelos, A.; Madrigal-Bujaidar, E.; de la Cruz, C. Inhibitory effect of chamomile essential oil on the sister chromatid exchanges induced by daunorubicin and methyl methanesulfonate in mouse bone marrow. *Toxicol. Lett.,* **2002**, *135*(1-2), 103-110.
[http://dx.doi.org/10.1016/S0378-4274(02)00253-9] [PMID: 12243869]

[69] Achterrath-Tuckermann, U.; Kunde, R.; Flaskamp, E.; Isaac, O.; Thiemer, K. [Pharmacological investigations with compounds of chamomile. V. Investigations on the spasmolytic effect of compounds of chamomile and Kamillosan on the isolated guinea pig ileum]. *Planta Med.,* **1980**, *39*(1), 38-50.
[http://dx.doi.org/10.1055/s-2008-1074901] [PMID: 7403307]

[70] Maliakal, P.P.; Wanwimolruk, S. Effect of herbal teas on hepatic drug metabolizing enzymes in rats. *J. Pharm. Pharmacol.,* **2010**, *53*(10), 1323-1329.
[http://dx.doi.org/10.1211/0022357011777819] [PMID: 11697539]

[71] Gupta, A.K.; Misra, N. Hepatoprotective Activity of Aqueous Ethanolic Extract of *Chamomile capitula* in Paracetamol Intoxicated Albino Rats. *Am. J. Pharmacol. Toxicol.,* **2006**, *1*(1), 17-20.
[http://dx.doi.org/10.3844/ajptsp.2006.17.20]

[72] Al-Hashem, F.H. Gastroprotective effects of aqueous extract of *Chamomilla recutita* against ethanol-induced gastric ulcers. *Saudi Med. J.,* **2010**, *31*(11), 1211-1216.
[PMID: 21063650]

[73] Aksoy, L.; Sözbilir, N.B. Effects of *Matricaria chamomilla L.* on lipid peroxidation, antioxidant enzyme systems, and key liver enzymes in CCl$_4$-treated rats. *Toxicol. Environ. Chem.,* **2012**, *94*(9), 1780-1788.
[http://dx.doi.org/10.1080/02772248.2012.729837]

[74] Hamid, S.; Sabir, A.; Khan, S.; Aziz, P. Experimental cultivation of *Silybum marianum* and chemical composition of its oil. *Pak. J. Sci. Ind. Res.,* **1983**, *26*, 244-246.

[75] Morazzoni, P.; Bombardelli, E. Silybum marianum & Cardusarianum. *Fitoterapia,* **1995**, *66*, 3-42.

[76] Lee, D.Y.W.; Liu, Y. Molecular structure and stereochemistry of silybin A, silybin B, isosilybin A,

and isosilybin B, Isolated from Silybum marianum (milk thistle). *J. Nat. Prod.,* **2003**, *66*(9), 1171-1174.
[http://dx.doi.org/10.1021/np030163b] [PMID: 14510591]

[77]   Ligeret, H.; Brault, A.; Vallerand, D.; Haddad, Y.; Haddad, P.S. Antioxidant and mitochondrial protective effects of silibinin in cold preservation–warm reperfusion liver injury. *J. Ethnopharmacol.,* **2008**, *115*(3), 507-514.
[http://dx.doi.org/10.1016/j.jep.2007.10.024] [PMID: 18061382]

[78]   Shaker, E.; Mahmoud, H.; Mnaa, S. Silymarin, the antioxidant component and *Silybum marianum* extracts prevent liver damage. *Food Chem. Toxicol.,* **2010**, *48*(3), 803-806.
[http://dx.doi.org/10.1016/j.fct.2009.12.011] [PMID: 20034535]

[79]   Abou Zid, S. Silymarin, natural flavonolignans from milk thistle. In: *Phytochemicals-A Global Perspective of Their Role in Nutrition and Health*; Venketeshwer, R., Ed.; Croatia InTech: Rijeka, **2012**; pp. 255-272.
[http://dx.doi.org/10.5772/26027]

[80]   Deep, G.; Oberlies, N.H.; Kroll, D.J.; Agarwal, R. Isosilybin B and isosilybin A inhibit growth, induce G1 arrest and cause apoptosis in human prostate cancer LNCaP and 22Rv1 cells. *Carcinogenesis,* **2007**, *28*(7), 1533-1542.
[http://dx.doi.org/10.1093/carcin/bgm069] [PMID: 17389612]

[81]   Svobodová, A.; Zdařilová, A.; Walterová, D.; Vostálová, J. Flavonolignans from *Silybum marianum* moderate UVA-induced oxidative damage to HaCaT keratinocytes. *J. Dermatol. Sci.,* **2007**, *48*(3), 213-224.
[http://dx.doi.org/10.1016/j.jdermsci.2007.06.008] [PMID: 17689055]

[82]   Hikino, H.; Kiso, Y.; Wagner, H.; Fiebig, M. Antihepatotoxic actions of flavonolignans from *Silybum marianum* fruits. *Planta Med.,* **1984**, *50*(3), 248-250.
[http://dx.doi.org/10.1055/s-2007-969690] [PMID: 6091165]

[83]   Flora, K.; Hahn, M.; Rosen, H.; Benner, K. Milk thistle (*Silybum marianum*) for the therapy of liver disease. *Am. J. Gastroenterol.,* **1998**, *93*(2), 139-143.
[http://dx.doi.org/10.1111/j.1572-0241.1998.00139.x] [PMID: 9468229]

SUBJECT INDEX

A

Acanthopleura vaillantii 66
Acanthosis nigricans 12
Acid(s) 4, 19, 20, 28, 29, 44, 50, 51, 56, 61, 63, 66, 67, 68, 71, 90, 100, 101, 134, 148, 149, 159, 163, 173
  ascorbic 90, 100
  betulinic 29
  bile 19, 20
  caffeoylquinic 51
  carnosic 29
  chebulinic 63, 68
  chlorogenic 29, 44, 50, 63, 66, 68, 71
  chtolphenolic 29
  coumaric 29, 66
  cryptochlorogenic 51
  dicaffeoylquinic 29
  echinocystic 29
  ellagic 28
  Ferulic 149
  folic 163
  fumaric 134, 148
  gallic 28, 29, 67
  glycyrrhizic 61, 65
  hexadecanoic 28
  hyaluronic 173
  hydroxycinnamic 51
  Ilicic 29
  neochlorogenic 51
  nicotinic 4
  oleanolic 29
  oleic 56
  phonic 62
  propenoic 28
  rosmarinic 29
  thiobarbituric 28, 93, 101
  trifluoroacetic 66, 159
  ursolic 29
Action 164, 171
  anticancer 171
  anti-inflammatory biological 164

Activating pro-apoptotic proteins 48
Acyl carrier protein (ACP) 93, 141, 142, 148
Adenine nucleotide translocator 32
Agents 4, 50, 61, 81, 100, 154, 163, 164
  allopathic 61
  anti-lipoperoxidation 50
  chemotherapeutic 81
  hepato-regenerative 100
Alanine aminotransferase 4, 148, 173
Alcoholic liver disease (ALD) 10, 12, 66, 100
Allium sativum 86, 96, 138
Aloe vera 29, 120
Amaranthus spinosus 44, 55, 71
Antioxidant enzymes 28, 46, 49, 51, 54, 56, 96, 101
  superoxide dismutase 101
Apoptosis 47, 48, 53, 54, 55, 57, 64, 66, 89, 149
  caspase-dependent 57
  hepatocyte 48
  protein 55
Arthritis, rheumatoid 163
Aspartate aminotransferase 48, 86, 148, 173
ATP energy 50
Atractyloside poisoning 32
Autoimmune illnesses 84
  inflammatory 84

B

Blood proteins 20
Brassica 139, 140, 147
  juncea 139
  oleracea 140, 147
Budd-Chiari syndrome 84

C

Camilla sinensis 167
Cancer 27, 32, 45, 69, 81, 84, 90, 168
  hepatic 90
  hepatocellular 27, 69, 81